MW00603812

Foundations
of Case Management

A Practical Guide for RNs Transitioning from Nurse to Case Manager

Deanna Cooper Gillingham, RN, CCM

Copyright © 2021 Deanna Cooper Gillingham

All rights reserved.

i

Foundations of Case Management is an independent publication and has not been authorized, or otherwise approved by the owners of the trademarks or organizations referred to in this product. The author is not affiliated with or endorsed by any organization. All names and acronyms are trademarks of their owners.

Although the author and publisher have made every effort to ensure that the information in this book was correct at press time, the author and publisher do not assume and hereby disclaim any liability to any party for any loss, damage, or disruption caused by errors or omissions, whether such errors or omissions result from negligence, accident, or any other cause.

Because of the dynamic nature of the Internet, any web addresses or links contained in this book may have changed since publication and may no longer be valid.

The author of this book does not dispense medical advice or prescribe the use of any technique as a form of treatment for physical, emotional, or medical problems without the advice of a physician, either directly or indirectly. The intent of the author is only to offer information.

Copyright © 2021 Deanna Cooper Gillingham

All rights reserved. No part of this book may be used or reproduced by any means, graphic, electronic, or mechanical, including photocopying, recording, taping or by any information storage retrieval system without the prior written permission of the publisher except in the case of brief quotations embodied in critical articles and reviews.

To request permission, contact the publisher at Info@BlueBayouPress.com

ISBN Paperback: 978-1-943889-15-0

Library of Congress Control Number: 2021918965

Edited by Blyss Splane

Cover art by Abigail Gusto

Interior Design by Andrea Morris

Excerpt from CMSA's Standards of Practice for Case Managers reprinted with permission, the Case Management Society of America, 6301 Ranch Drive, Little Rock, AR 72223, www.cmsa.org.

Published in the United States by HCP2HCP an imprint of Blue Bayou Press, LLC, Crestview, FL 32536

BlueBayouPress.com

DEDICATION

This book is dedicated to Richard Culliver. In your short time on this planet you managed to bring tremendous joy and inspiration to so many people, including me. You continue to inspire me every day and live on in our hearts.

ACKNOWLEDGEMENTS

The number of people involved in bringing this book to fruition is as large as the number of stars in the sky. Every case manager who has shaped the practice of case management should be included. But since I can't do that, I will acknowledge a few of the people who have directly helped this book come to life.

Lois May, Marty Pressley-Turner, Anne Llewellyn, Ellen Fink-Samnick, Colleen Morley, Julie Castine, Barbara Kuritz, and Abi Carmen.

I also want to thank each one of you who asked for this book. Without your requests and encouragement, it would still be a work in progress.

Contents

Part 1: Introduction to Case Management   1

Contents

Contents

Contents

Contents

Contents

Contents

Contents

Contents

Contents

Contents

Introduction

Congratulations on your decision to advance your career and become a case manager! It seems like not that long ago, I was in your shoes, transitioning from a more traditional nursing role to case management. I remember the nervousness and uncertainty I felt taking on this new role when I really didn't understand the role of case management.

I also remember reading books about case management that left me feeling more confused and uncertain. I felt like I was back in school and entered the class late. They were using terminology I didn't fully understand and discussing concepts that were foreign to me. I realized that the foundations of case management were missing.

With some great mentoring, I was able to fumble my way through my first year as a case manager (thank you Tammy Blachura, Marty Pressly-Turner, Brenda El Dada, and the Lunch Bunch). It took six months before I was finally able to explain the role of a case manager. Six months! I was told this was normal. I can still remember thinking there has got to be a better way.

Fast forward years later and there still isn't a better way. I decided to create what was missing: the book I wanted when I started in this specialty. The book that would explain how to take the knowledge and skills you have acquired as a nurse to successfully transition into case management. The book that teaches what case management is and how to practice case management with excellence.

Like my previous book, *CCM Certification Made Easy: Your Guide to Passing the Certified Case Manager Exam*, this book contains no filler or fluff, just what you need to know to successfully begin working as a case manager. It is presented in a way that is easy to read and understand.

A few things you should know before diving in...

You will notice that we use the word "client" most of the time when referring to the person we are working with. When working in an acute care setting, we are used to referring to this person as the patient. In the insurance setting, this person is known as a member. While you may see both of these terms used in this book, we prefer to use the term "client."

The term "patient" implies someone who is ill or injured and needs someone to care for them. Psychologically, it puts us in a position of power while disempowering the other person. The term "client" implies that the case manager is working for and with them.

To avoid using he/she all of the time, we have chosen to be consistent in using *he* for the client/patient/member, and *she* for the case manager. We understand that there are male and non-binary nurses and case managers, as there are female and non-binary clients. This decision was made solely for ease of reading and for clarity between the case manager and patient.

Take the Foundations of Case Management Course and get nursing CE credit!

Did you know that there is a course you can take that follows along with this book? After completing the course you will receive a certificate of completion from the Case Management Institute that you can proudly add to your resume and LinkedIn profile.

In addition, the course provides you with:

- Nursing CE
- Assignments to solidify your learning
- Individualized instructor support and feedback on your assignments to ensure you "get it"
- Access to the best case management instructors in the industry!

For more information go to:

CaseManagementInstitute.com

Part 1: Introduction to Case Management

Outcomes

Readers will be able to:

- Explain what case management is, as well as the philosophy and Goals of case management practice.

- Identify times in their nursing practice where they have performed activities that are transferable to case management.

- Identify the roles, functions, and activities the case manager performs.

- Explain how the functions and activities of the case manager will vary based on the work setting.

- Compare the different case management models used in the inpatient setting.

- Assess each case management model's strengths and weaknesses.

- Identify the skills and qualities that need to be developed to be a competent case manager.

- Rate her level of competence with each of the required skills and/or qualities of case managers.

- Assess her ability to work as a competent case manager.

Part 1: Introduction to Case Management

Chapter 1

Definition, Philosophy, and Goals of Case Management

Definitions of Case Management

The Commission for Case Manager Certification (CCMC) defines case management as

> a collaborative process that assesses, plans, implements, coordinates, monitors, and evaluates the options and services required to meet the client's health and human services needs. It is characterized by advocacy, communication, and resource management and promotes quality and cost-effective interventions and outcomes" (Definition and philosophy of case management I Commission for Case Manager Certification (CCMC), 2017).

Let's break this down and look at what this definition means.

"A collaborative process": Case management is performed in collaboration with many stakeholders, including but not limited to the client, their family and/or support system, physicians, pharmacists, and other members of the healthcare team.

"That assesses": Case managers perform initial and ongoing assessments with their clients to identify their client's goals, any potential or actual barriers that may interfere with the client reaching their goals, and any barriers to following the treatment plan. Case managers continue to assess on an ongoing basis to identify new barriers that may arise. This assessment is an essential part of case management, and the reason CCMC requires a license or certification that allows the professional to conduct an assessment independently within the scope of practice to become a Certified Case Manager (CCM).

"Plans": Once the client has been assessed, the case manager (CM) develops a plan in collaboration with other stakeholders to resolve identified issues, barriers, or potential barriers. The client is always involved in creating this plan, as without their buy-in, the plan is not likely to succeed.

"Implements": This is where the plan that was created is carried out.

"Coordinates": The CM coordinates the services (ex: durable medical equipment (DME), home care), and resources (ex: community and/or financial resources) used in the client's treatment and care.

"Monitors and evaluates": The CM monitors and evaluates the client's progress, the effectiveness of the treatment plan, progress made toward achieving the client's goals, and the items that were implemented and coordinated during those respective phases.

"The options and services required to meet the client's health and human service needs": Case management involves whole client care. CMs understand that the health of a person does not occur in a vacuum and therefore address the human services, as well as the healthcare resources available to the client.

"It is characterized by advocacy": CMs are primarily patient advocates, regardless of the setting where they work. The primary focus of everything we do must have the best interests of the patient, as the patient sees it, at the center.

Communication": Communication plays a major role in case management. The CM must communicate effectively with the client as well as other stakeholders. Utilizing strong communication skills is a competency all CMs must strive to meet.

"...and resource management and promotes quality and cost-effective interventions and outcomes": In this day and age, when health care costs are spiraling out of control and adequate healthcare is out of reach for many Americans, resource management has become an important issue. CMs find a variety of ways to ensure the appropriate use of resources, which ultimately reduces the cost of the client's care. These include but are not limited to, ensuring the appropriate level of care, timeliness of services, and maintaining the quality of care.

CMSA in their 2016 Standards of Practice updated their definition of case management to read:

> Case Management is a collaborative process of assessment, planning, facilitation, care coordination, evaluation and advocacy for options and services to meet an

individual's and family's comprehensive health needs through communication and available resources to promote patient safety, quality of care, and cost-effective outcomes (Case Management Society of America, 2016).

There are some subtle differences in these definitions, and CMSA has added "promotion of patient safety" to their definition, but as you can see, they have the same general idea. So now that we know the definition of case management, let's talk about what CMs do.

So, What Does A Case Manager Do?

The activities of a CM will change depending on the setting where they are working. We will take a deep dive into all the roles and functions of CMs a little later. For now, know that CMs rarely, if ever provide hands-on patient care (there are exceptions to this that will be covered later). Rather, CMs guide their clients in discovering their goals related to their health and healthcare, and then help them to reach those goals. The rewards in case management come from helping clients and their families address problems so that they can transition through the complex healthcare system in a dignified manner and move on with their life, or sometimes their death.

Much of what case managers do to help clients solve problems and transition through the healthcare system revolves around education, patient advocacy, and care coordination.

CMs provide ongoing education to the client and their families regarding the plan of care, treatment options, medication management, discharge instructions, disease management, and community resources, to name a few. CMs act as a patient advocate, ensuring the patient's best interests are at the forefront of every decision. They advocate by providing education to other healthcare and service providers to understand and respect the goals and needs of the client.

Care coordination is another important part of case management. CMs ensure the right care is provided in the right setting and in a timely manner. They coordinate care by multiple providers, arrange for delivery of care, and ensure safe transitions in care.

Philosophy and Guiding Principles

To really understand what CMs do, you must understand the philosophy and guiding principles behind case management. The Case Management Society of America (CMSA) covers these in their *Standards of Practice for Case Management* in section IV, Philosophy and Guiding Principles.

Please note that at the time of this writing, CMSA is currently in the process of updating the Standards of Practice, and the 2016 Standards of Practice are the most current. Please contact CMSA for more information on the update.

IV. Philosophy and Guiding Principles

A. Statement of Philosophy

A philosophy is a statement of belief and values that sets forth principles to guide a program, its meaning, its context, and the role of the individual(s) that exist in it. The CMSA's philosophy of case management articulates that:

- The underlying premise of case management is based in the fact that, when an individual reaches the optimum level of wellness and functional capability, everyone benefits: the individual client being served, the client's family or family caregiver, the health care delivery system, the reimbursement source or payer, and other involved parties such as the employer and consumer advocates.

- Professional case management serves as a means for achieving client wellness and autonomy through advocacy, ongoing communication, health education, identification of service resources, and service facilitation.

- Professional case management services are best offered in a climate that allows client's engagement and direct communication among the case manager, the client, the client's family or family caregiver, and appropriate service personnel, in order to optimize health outcomes for all concerned (CMSA, 2009).

The philosophy of case management underscores the recommendation that at-risk individuals, especially those with complex medical, behavioral, and/or psychosocial needs, be evaluated for case management intervention. The key philosophical components of case management address care that is holistic and client-centered, with mutual goals, allowing stewardship of resources for the client and the health care system including the diverse group of stakeholders. Through these efforts, case management focuses simultaneously on achieving optimal health and attaining wellness to the highest level possible for each client.

It is the philosophy of case management that when the provision of health care is effective and efficient, all parties benefit. Case management, provided as part of a collabo- rative and interprofessional health care team, serves to identify options and resources which are acceptable to the client and client's family or family caregiver. This then, in turn, increases the potential for effective client's engagement in self-management, adherence to the case management plan of care, and the achievement of successful outcomes.

Case management interventions focus on improving care coordination and reducing the fragmentation of the services the recipients of care often experience especially when multiple health care providers and different care settings are involved. Taken collectively, case management interventions are intended to enhance client safety, well-being, and quality of life. These interventions carefully consider health care costs through the professional case manager's recommendations of cost-effective and efficient alternatives for care. Thus, effective case management directly and positively impacts the health care delivery system especially in realizing the goals of the "Triple Aim" which include improving the health outcomes of individuals and populations, enhancing the experience of health care, and reducing the cost of care.

B. Guiding Principles

Guiding principles are relevant and meaningful concepts that clarify or guide practice. Guiding principles for case management practice provide that professional case managers:

- Use a client-centric, collaborative part-nership approach that is responsive to the individual client's culture, preferences, needs, and values.

- Facilitate client's self-determination and self-management through the tenets of ad- vocacy, shared and informed decision-mak- ing, counseling, and health education, whenever possible.

- Use a comprehensive, holistic, and com-passionate approach to care delivery which integrates a client's medical, behavioral, social, psychological, functional, and other needs.

- Practice cultural and linguistic sensitivity, and maintain current knowledge of diverse populations within their practice demo-graphics.

- Implement evidence-based care guidelines in the care of clients, as available and appli-cable to the practice setting and/or client population served.

- Promote optimal client safety at the individ-ual, organizational, and community level.

- Promote the integration of behavioral change science and principles throughout the case management process.

- Facilitate awareness of and connections with community supports and resources.

- Foster safe and manageable navigation through the health care system to enhance the client's timely access to services and the achievement of successful outcomes.

- Pursue professional knowledge and practice excellence and maintain competence in case management and health and human service delivery.

- Support systematic approaches to quality management and health outcomes im-provement, implementation of practice in-novations, and dissemination of knowledge and practice to the health care community.

- Maintain compliance with federal, state, and local rules and regulations, and orga-nizational, accreditation, and certification standards.

- Demonstrate knowledge, skills, and compe-tency in the application of case manage-ment standards of practice and relevant codes of ethics and professional conduct.

Case management guiding principles, interventions, and strategies target the achievement of optimal wellness, function, and autonomy for the client and client's family or family caregiver through advocacy, assessment, planning, communication, health education, resource management, care coordination, collaboration, and service facilitation.

The professional case manager applies these principles into practice based on the individualized needs and values of the client to assure, in collaboration with the interprofessional health care team, the provision of safe, appropri-ate, effective, client-centered, timely, efficient, and equitable care and services.

Excerpt from CMSA's Standards of Practice for Case Managers. *Reprinted with permission, the Case Management Society of America, 6301 Ranch Drive, Little Rock, AR 72223, www.cmsa.org.*

Part 1: Introduction to Case Management

Chapter 2

The Case Manager's Roles, Functions, and Activities

Defining Role, Function, and Activity

Let's start by defining the terms *role*, *function*, and *activity*. An activity is an action or task that is done. A function is a group of related actions or tasks that combine to form a function. And a role is the function assumed or part played by a person or thing in a particular situation. Note how they build on each other. The role of the CM includes but is not limited to playing the part of a patient advocate, an educator, and a facilitator.

Many case management activities and functions are the same regardless of setting, such as advocacy, assessment, planning, empowerment, facilitation, collaboration, and education. For example, all CMs conduct comprehensive assessments of the client's needs. From the assessment, a case management plan is developed in collaboration with the client and family.

All CMs collaborate with the client and his or her family, caregiver, physician, provider, and/or payer to achieve high-quality, cost-efficient outcomes. This requires the CM to facilitate communication and coordination between all members involved in the client's care. She must also educate the client, family, and members of the healthcare team regarding treatment options, insurance benefits, and community resources to facilitate informed decision-making. This empowers the client and promotes self-advocacy.

Every CM must advocate for the client as one of the main functions of the role. The goal is to achieve the best outcome for the client, provider, and payer. If a conflict arises, the client's needs take priority. It is important to remember your role as a patient advocate is to always advocate in the best interest of the client.

Case in Point

Stephen is a 7-year-old recently diagnosed with an inoperable brain tumor. His ability to ambulate has deteriorated quickly and he is now unable to stand or walk, even with an assistive device. You work at the pediatric oncologist's office as his case manager. Because Stephen is a minor you are working with his mother, Renee.

During a follow-up call, Renee states she is now having to carry Stephen, which is resulting in back pain for her. At a support group meeting she attends for parents of children with cancer, one of the other moms had a large stroller for her daughter. Renee would like one of these for Stephen and would like your assistance in obtaining it. You agree to discuss it with Stephen's oncologist, who will need to write the order.

Two days later Renee calls to tell you the request for the stroller has been denied. You agree to contact the insurance company on her behalf. You find out that the Medical Director denied the request because the stroller does not qualify as durable medical equipment (DME). To qualify as DME the item has to be medical equipment and this stroller does not fall into that category. They will, however, pay for a wheelchair for Stephen. You proceed to inform both Renee and the physician of this information and facilitate obtaining a wheelchair for Stephen.

A pediatric wheelchair is obtained for Stephen. On a follow-up phone call, Renee states that although she appreciates the wheelchair and it does help, she would still like the stroller. The wheelchair is large, heavy, and cumbersome. It is difficult to travel with because of its size. One of Renee's goals for Stephen is that he gets to experience a lifetime of adventures in the limited time he has remaining on earth, and she feels the stroller would make this easier.

You discuss this with the physician and the decision is made to appeal the denial for the stroller. The physician requests a peer-to-peer review with the insurance company Medical Director in an attempt to get the denial overturned.

Unfortunately, the peer-to-peer review does not result in the denial being overturned. The Medical Director is bound by the insurance contract, which states only medical equipment is covered by the policy.

You inform Renee of the decision and reassure her that you will continue to look at options for obtaining the stroller. You assess her ability to contribute to the cost of the stroller. You find that her FMLA ran out last month and she lost her job because as Stephen's full-time caregiver, she is no longer able to work.

After a week of searching, you are finally able to come up with a way to get Stephen and Renee the stroller. You have found a stroller that is very similar to the one Renee originally wanted. It has all the features she needs and is only $997. You have also found a charitable organization that provides $1000 grants for families of children with terminal cancer to use for anything not covered by insurance. You connect Renee to the organization and she fills out the application. Two weeks later she receives her stroller.

This Case In Point is a reminder that as the case manager, our job is not to "get the insurance company to pay" for something. Rather, our goal is to help the client reach their goal(s). When traditional methods are exhausted, it is our job to look at creative alternatives.

Case Management Settings and Related Functions

While this book focuses on nurse CMs, it is important to note that there are CMs from other health and human service disciplines. Nurses and social workers make up the majority of CMs, but pharmacists, physical therapists, occupational therapists, speech therapists, respiratory therapists, and many other disciplines add a valuable dimension to the profession of case management.

Some functions of the CM will vary based on the practice setting, the complexity of the population served, and her professional discipline (registered nurse, social worker, disability manager, rehabilitation counselor, physical therapist, etc.). As the role of the CM changes based on these factors, so do their functions and activities.

The setting where the CM works plays a large part in determining the actions and functions performed, and the extent to which each of these is carried out. We will look at the various case management settings and the functions and activities associated with each setting.

Ambulatory care settings

Such as physician's offices, ambulatory care clinics, accountable care organizations, corporations, and community-based organizations, including healthcare centers, schools, and university clinics.

CMs in these settings may focus on the general population, on high-risk populations, or both. These roles are geared toward prevention and providing education and support to empower individuals to keep or reach their optimal level of health and wellness.

Activities may include:
- Running wellness and screening programs
- Providing health risk assessments
- Assessing social determinants of health
- Implementing risk-reduction strategies
- Assisting with disease management
- Triaging over the phone
- Facilitating access to services
- Referring to community-based resources
- Coordinating medical and social services
- Ensuring patient knowledge and compliance with treatment
- Monitoring clients
- Providing education

Acute and sub-acute care settings

Such as hospitals, acute inpatient rehabilitation, long term acute care hospitals (LTACH), and skilled nursing facilities (SNF)

The roles in these organizations are focused on cost-effective care in the appropriate setting that meets guidelines for reimbursement while providing safe transitions and discharge planning.

Activities may include:

- Verification of benefits
- Authorization of services
- Utilization review
- Discharge planning
- Resource management
- Coordination of care among team members
- Coordinate interdisciplinary team (ICT) meetings
- Facilitate referrals
- Transitions of care
- Goal planning with patient and family

Managed care/payer-based settings

Such as public health insurance programs (Medicare, Medicaid, state-funded programs) and private health insurance programs (occupational health, disability, group health insurance, managed care organizations).

Case management in these types of organizations focuses on utilization management and education.

Activities may include:

- Acting as a liaison between providers, members, and insurance company
- Coordinating care
- Promoting high-quality care
- Negotiating for services
- Monitoring for compliance with the treatment plan
- Ensuring the appropriate level of care and care setting
- Informing clients about healthcare benefits
- Educating clients
- Utilization management
- Discharge planning

Palliative care, home care, and hospice care

Case managers in these settings combine the role of the hands-on nurse with the case manager.

Activities may include:

- Liaise with providers
- Communicate with treating physicians
- Provide patient and family education
- Assess for and coordinate additional services and DME
- Provide skilled nursing care
- Coordinate interdisciplinary care team meetings

Workers' Compensation organizations

Case management in Workers' Compensation cases focuses on vocational activities, such as collaborating with the employer to get the employee back to work.

Activities may include:

- Coordinate care between multiple healthcare providers
- Facilitate communication between the employer, claims adjuster, attorneys, union representative, state administrative agency, and providers
- Monitor client progress
- Utilization review
- Obtain precertification when necessary
- Obtain job analysis
- Accompany injured workers during physician appointments
- Help the injured worker understand the benefits of the coverage and the requirements for the patient
- Educate the injured worker about their injury and explain the work comp system they are under
- Assist with additional resources if not covered under WC benefits

Chapter 3

Case Management Models

Introduction

In the inpatient setting, there are many different models of case management. When interviewing for an inpatient CM position, you will want to ask about the case management model in use at that facility. This information will give you a good idea of what the roles and responsibilities will be for each team member.

For those not working in an inpatient setting, it is still helpful to understand the various models. At some point, you will most likely be working in collaboration with a hospital or other inpatient case management department. Learning about the different models will help you collaborate with the correct team members for various purposes.

We will look at the three most common models that each have the following three roles.

(1) Patient-flow - Ensuring the patient moves through the acute care setting in a timely manner

(2) Utilization Management (UM) - Communicating with payer sources

(3) Discharge Planning (DCP) - Moving the patient to the next level of care. This includes assessing for any needs the patient may have after they leave the acute care setting while ensuring the safe, timely, and appropriate discharge with appropriate resources.

Common Case Management Models

Integrated Case Management Model

Integrated CM Model - All roles (patient flow, UM, and DCP) are performed by a single nurse CM. In this model, a social worker may be consulted when appropriate.

The person who carries out these three roles is what differentiates each model. While there are additional models, most are a variation of one of the following models.

Dyad Model

Dyad Model - RN and social work case managers work together in one department. They may co-manage the client with divided responsibilities. The RN provides education and addresses clinical issues. The SW focuses on financial, social, and discharge needs. Alternatively, either role may perform an initial assessment, and after determining the primary needs of the client (medical vs. social), one person would take on the responsibility for the client with the other available as a resource.

Triad Model

Triad Model / Collaborative Case Management (UM/CM/SW) - This model is similar to the Dyad Model, but a third person is involved who takes over the UM activities working with the third-party payer. This leaves the RN and SW CMs to focus on patient flow, transitions, and DCP.

Strengths and Weaknesses of Models

There are strengths and weaknesses to all of these models. For example, with the integrated model, the CM really knows the details of the case. She is in direct communication with the payer, vendors, patient, physicians, and other staff. This reduces duplication and fragmentation of care, which may be more cost-effective and time-efficient. On the other hand, it is more time-consuming and requires adequate staffing.

The Collaborative Model eliminates the very time-consuming UM task for the CM. This allows the CM to focus on other functions for the client. It requires strong and clear communication between the team members, and this model works best if all team members are in the same department and report to the same supervisor. There can also be some redundancy with this model, such as assessments and chart review.

Chapter 4

Required Skills and Qualities of the Case Manager

Introduction

Case management is not for everyone. Without the skills and qualities necessary for case management, it's possible you will detest your job and your clients will suffer. Certain skills can be developed, such as organization, time management, and computer skills. However, many of the qualities that make a good CM are intrinsic. For example, without the strong, innate desire to advocate for your client, you will not see the importance of opportunities to do so. This inevitably results in poor client outcomes and poor job performance.

Skills for Case Managers

Experience

Case managers need a thorough understanding of how the healthcare system works in practice, not just theory. For this reason, a firm clinical foundation is essential for success. The consensus is that a minimum of five years of healthcare industry experience, mostly in acute care, is necessary for someone entering the field of case management. Case management is not an entry-level position, but rather an area of expertise that requires the knowledge and skills that are accumulated and mastered over years in the practice setting.

Excellent communication skills

Excellent communication is an essential part of case management. Communication is how we conduct our assessments, advocate, negotiate, document, educate, and transition our clients. Without good communication skills, a CM cannot be successful. CMs need to communicate respectfully and effectively with all members of the healthcare team, the client, their family, and other stakeholders.

It is important for CMs to understand verbal and non-verbal communication, while listening carefully to hear both what is being said and what is not said. CMs also need to listen with an open mind to understand and practice empathic listening—considering the other person's perspective or frame of reference (values, beliefs, and feelings).

Interviewing skills

Interviewing skills are the ability to develop a rapport with the client that allows him to feel safe opening up and providing you with the information you need, including sensitive information. The CM needs to obtain needed information during the client interview, as this is the foundation for the remainder of the case management process. For this reason, good interview skills are a must.

Strong computer skills

Today's CM must have strong computer skills. The RN case manager replaces her stethoscope with a computer. The computer is used for client selection, a portion of the assessment, documentation, research, and communication.

Basic proficiency in the use of Microsoft Word, Excel, and Outlook Mail is necessary for most case management positions. CMs must also have basic computer skills to build on that will allow them to learn how to use new computer software to send and retrieve information and documentation, determine the length of stay, and document.

Examples of how CMs use computers:
- Software that finds clients at high risk who may benefit from case management services
- Access to the client's medical record
- Documentation of assessment, intervention, response, and communication
- Researching unfamiliar diseases and available community resources

- Utilizing Google or other search engines for information and resources
- Prioritization, organization, and time management skills

CMs are busy people. To get everything done they need excellent prioritization, organization, and time management skills that enable them to work quickly and efficiently. CMs will have a variety of tasks to perform, making it necessary to prioritize those tasks and manage their time wisely. Organizational skills will help them find the resources they need to do their job quickly.

Qualities for Case Managers

Adaptability/flexibility

Things are always changing. It's good to start the day with a plan, but things will come up, and CMs need to be flexible and adaptable to change when this happens.

Independent worker, but knows when to ask for help

CMs MUST be able to work independently. They need to know what needs to be done and how to do it. There will always be an occasion where the help of others is needed, and CMs must be willing to ask for help in these scenarios. For day-to-day work as a CM, you are expected to perform your role autonomously without direction.

The ability to problem-solve/critical thinking skills

Critical thinking involves reasoning, organizing, and analyzing information so that problems are understood and appropriate solutions are developed. CMs often get a large amount of information and need to determine what is relevant. They need to understand the problem(s) or potential problem(s), and then formulate and implement a plan that will resolve or prevent the problem(s).

Strong interpersonal skills

Interpersonal skills are the ability to communicate and interact with others. CMs do not work in a vacuum; they are constantly collaborating with others. It's essential to be the type of person others enjoy working with to be an effective CM. You can't do your job if others are avoiding you because of a lack of interpersonal skills.

Ethics, values, integrity, and trust

These are a core part of case management and are covered in CMSA's Standards of Practice. These are non-negotiable traits for those entering case management.

Unrelenting advocacy

CMs must have both the desire and ability to advocate for the needs of the client. This includes conveying the client's desires to providers, caregivers, and family, as well as teaching self-advocacy to the client.

Compassion

Compassion refers to both an understanding of another's pain and more importantly for CMs, the desire to somehow mitigate that pain. It motivates the CM to want to go out of their way to help the physical, mental, or emotional pains of another. Without compassion, the CM will find themselves dreading going to work each day. They will also not be able to truly meet the needs of their client. CMs need to have the ability to have compassion for their clients, as well as other stakeholders.

Personal development

CMs need to be constantly learning so that they can best serve and educate their clients. Congratulations! By reading this book you are proving that you are committed to your personal development.

References

Chapter 1

Case Management Society of America. (2016). *Standards of Practice for Case Management* (pp. 12, 13, 27–28). Case Management Society of America.

Definition and philosophy of case management | Commission for Case Manager Certification (CCMC). (2017). ccmcertification.org; Commission for Case Management Certification. https://ccmcertification.org/about-ccmc/about-case-management/definition-and-philosophy-case-management

Part 1: Introduction to Case Management

Part 2: The Case Management Process

Outcomes

Readers will be able to:

- List the components of the case management process
- Compare the case management process to the nursing process
- Explain how the case management process is nonlinear
- Describe the types of patients who benefit from case management
- Compare the case management assessment to the nursing assessment
- Describe the importance of the initial case management assessment
- Demonstrate techniques to complete the client assessment accurately, completely, and in a timely manner
- List the steps to facilitating a successful initial assessment interview
- Describe medication reconciliation per The Joint Commission guidelines
- Apply medication reconciliation to client cases
- Explain the goal of medication reconciliation
- Identify the assessment tools available to screen clients for health literacy, depression, substance abuse, and functioning
- Describe the objective of the planning phase of the case management process
- Create SMART goals with client input
- Explain the importance of client involvement in creating the case management plan of care
- Explain the case manager's role during the implementation phase of the case management plan of care
- Explain the case manager's responsibilities during the monitoring and evaluation phase of the case management plan of care
- List reasons for closing a client to case management services
- Explain anylegal ramifications of terminating case management services

Part 2: The Case Management Process

Chapter 5

Introduction to the Case Management Process

Overview of the Case Management Process

The nursing profession utilizes the nursing process, AD PIE, which stands for:
- Assessment
- Diagnosis
- Planning/Outcomes
- Implementation
- Evaluation

Case management uses the case management process, which includes:
- Selection/Screening
- Assessment
- Planning
- Implementation
- Monitoring
- Closure

Unlike the nursing process, the case management process does not have a standard across the industry. Depending on the source, there can be fewer or additional phases and possibly different names for the phases. The process is the same, but some literature combines multiple phases into one phase, while others list them as separate and distinct phases. We will talk about the six-phase process.

It is important to note that these phases occur and reoccur in cycles, and they are not unidirectional or sequential. This means that CMs do not complete a phase and check it off their list. Many phases will take place concurrently or be revisited and repeated. For example, a new problem may arise during a follow-up with a patient. The CM would then return to the planning phase for that problem while continuing to follow up on the original problem. (See Figure 5-1.)

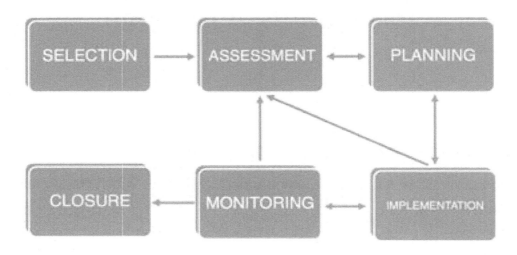

Figure 5-1. The Case Management Process.

The case management process revolves around the client and their support systems. It treats the client holistically, addressing the medical, physical, emotional, financial, psychosocial, behavioral, and other needs of the client as well as those of their support systems (*Case management philosophy and guiding principles | CCMC's case management body of knowledge (CMBOK)*, n.d.).

The case management process is adaptive to the various settings where CMs practice, as well as the settings where clients receive health and human services (*Case management philosophy and guiding principles | CCMC's case management body of knowledge (CMBOK)*, n.d.).

Chapter 6

Step One of the Case Management Process

Client Identification, Selection, and Engagement for Case Management Services

Stratifying risk

Potential clients may be introduced to the case manager in a variety of ways, including:

- Software that identifies high risk, high utilization, or high-cost individuals based on numerous factors (e.g., diagnosis, high dollar claims, polypharmacy, and/or frequent hospitalization or ER visits)
- Admission to a facility or unit within a facility
- Referrals by other professionals
- Self-referral

Each case management program will have its own policies and procedures to determine how client referrals are received, risk-stratified, the qualifications to enter the program, and the selection process. When the referral comes in, the CM or other designated person will document the referral source, screen the client for appropriateness of case management services, and record the findings of the screening.

Screening

Not every potential client is appropriate for case management services. The CM or another designated person will screen the referred client to determine whether or not they are suitable for, and would benefit from, the case management program. This is done by reviewing the patient information available, contacting the potential client, and/ or contacting the referral source. Details obtained may include claims information, utilization of healthcare services, current health status, insurance eligibility, support systems, health history, and other factors that identify that the client is at risk.

Depending on the case management setting and type of services provided, some of the reasons clients may be appropriate for case management include:

- New diagnosis of a chronic, complex, or terminal condition
- Catastrophic or life-altering condition
- High-risk pregnancy
- High-dollar diagnosis or injury
- End-of-life care
- Barriers to accessing care and/or services
- Nonadherence to health regimens
- Poor health self-management
- High utilization (multiple admissions or emergency room visits)
- Lack of a primary care provider (PCP)
- Financial challenges
- Social issues, such as weak or nonexistent support system or lack of caregiver
- Lack of understanding of disease process and/or low health literacy
- Multiple providers
- Numerous transitions of care
- Polypharmacy
- Poor pain control
- Difficult discharge planning

Documentation

Once the individual is screened and identified as someone who would benefit from case management services, the CM will obtain consent for case management services as per their employer's policies. Hospital case management is generally understood to be covered under the consent for treatment form signed upon hospitalization. Some states do not require consent in Workers' Compensation case management, but this is changing. Even if your employer does not require written consent for case management services, it is best practice and part of CMSA's Standards of Practice to obtain informed consent for case management services. (*Case Management Society of America*, 2016). This can be done verbally or in writing and is to be documented in the client record.

Part 2: The Case Management Process

Chapter 7

Step Two of the Case Management Process

Comprehensive Assessment and Opportunity Identification

Once we have identified the client as someone who would benefit from case management services, we will move on to the comprehensive case management assessment. This is where information is gathered to help us manage the client's case, as well as identify additional needs and barriers.

A comprehensive, individualized, and client-centered needs-based assessment is conducted and documented when the case is opened. This assessment covers the client's health, physical, functional, psychological, behavioral, sexual, and social status and needs. It is not the traditional hands-on nursing assessment, but rather it is conducted by discussions with clients, health care providers, and a review of the medical records available. This assessment is based on the CM's practice setting and is used to identify the client's problems, needs, and interests. Once the data is collected, it is analyzed and used to develop a client-centered case management plan of care.

The assessment can be done in person or telephonically. In addition to speaking with the client, information can also be obtained from family, caregivers, providers, medical records, insurance representatives, the client's employer, and other sources. It is important to note you can *receive* information from family, caregivers, and others, but to *give* information you need permission from the client. This should be written consent when possible, following the HIPAA guidelines of your employer. Verbal consent can be obtained but needs to be obtained with each communication. When dealing with other healthcare providers, it is safe to relay information for "continuity of care" in most instances. Always follow the policies and procedures of your employer.

The initial assessment is similar to the screening. In fact, some of the information from the screening can be transferred to the assessment, but this initial assessment is much more comprehensive and provides a more in-depth look into the client's healthcare and overall situation. CMs understand that health and wellness involve much more than medical care. There are social, psychological, financial, cultural, and spiritual factors to consider when helping a client achieve optimal health and wellness.

It will be time-consuming and overwhelming for new CMs to complete the assessment because it is comprehensive and involves so many areas. With time and experience, CMs will develop the techniques and flow needed to complete the assessment accurately, completely, and in a timely manner. Some of these techniques include using open-ended questions and guided discussions that lead the conversation, bundling questions from different parts of the assessment that relate to each other, and going deeper with statements like "tell me more about…"

The assessment should not be done in a "check-off box" type of manner. This interaction establishes the CM's relationship with the client. Effective communication skills and open-ended questions get beyond the surface level and dig deep into the client's situation and needs. Due to the length of time it takes to complete the initial assessment, it may need to be broken up into more than one interaction for complex clients.

During this assessment, the CM is identifying needs, barriers, and gaps in care that will be addressed during the course of case management. She is also discovering what is important to the client to ensure a plan of care specific to that client can be developed.

The assessment may include but is not limited to…

Medical assessment:
- Current health status
- Current medical conditions
- Current medications including prescribed, over the counter (OTC), and supplements
- Medication management and adherence
- Medical/surgical history
- Treatment history including complementary or alternative medicine
- Nutritional status

- Treating physicians including PCP
- Past and current healthcare service utilization
- Health goals

Behavioral and Cognitive assessment:
- History of or current substance use or abuse
- Depression risk screening
- Cognitive functioning
- Health literacy
- Knowledge of health conditions and plan of care
- Adherence to the plan of care
- Self-care and self-management capability
- Readiness to change
- Engagement
- Health activation level

Social Assessment:
- Family dynamics
- Caregiver availability
- Community involvement and support (church, neighbor, friends, clubs)
- Support system
- Environment (living conditions, structure, neighborhood)
- Education
- Vocational status (employed, unemployed, retired, type of employment)
- Financial status including income and resources
- Socioeconomic background
- Access and availability of nutritious food

Housing
- Safety (living conditions, history of abuse and neglect, self-care, and functional ability)
- Access to care including health insurance, transportation, providers (identify barriers)
- Cultural values, beliefs
- Spiritual beliefs and values

- Sexuality, including how the client identifies
- Language preference
- Hobbies, interests, and activities
- Advance directive documentation

Functional assessment:

- Functional status (activities of daily living (ADLs) and instrumental activities of daily living (IADLs))

While some of the data to complete the initial assessment may be obtained from medical records, the client interview is the primary manner for obtaining information about the client to create an effective case management plan of care. It is imperative that the information obtained be complete and accurate. Therefore, it is critical that the CM has good interview skills. The following steps can be taken to facilitate a successful interview.

The Client Interview

Preparation

The interview should be scheduled for a time when there are no anticipated interruptions for either the client or the CM. When scheduling the interview, the CM should let the client know approximately how much time to allow and what information will be required. For example: "Mr. Smith, we will take approximately 60 minutes and will need a list of your current medications, as well as the names and contact information of your physicians."

Before the interview, review available information from the client's chart, medical records, prior encounters, etc. Again, the reviewed materials are not a substitute for the client interview.

Prevent interruptions or distractions by silencing cell phones, turning off the TV, closing the door, or any other appropriate action. If the interview is over the telephone, make sure the client is at a location where he will be comfortable talking about private health information. For example, if he is talking on a cell phone at the grocery store, arrange a time when the client will have more privacy. If the interview is in person, it should be held in a place that is private and allows the client to talk without being heard by others. The CM should sit near the client at an angle and level that will allow for eye contact.

Introduction

The CM should introduce herself, including her title and employer. For example, an insurance CM should reveal to the client that she works for the insurance company and then explain her role, and inform the patient about the purpose of the interview. The CM should ask the patient how he would like to be addressed. It is also a good idea to inform the client why there will be numerous questions asked.

Establish Rapport

Create an environment that helps the client feel safe disclosing sensitive, personal information. He will feel more comfortable disclosing personal information, health history, problems, and concerns after a positive rapport has been established. Smiling and showing authentic interest in the client as a human being by asking questions about his job, family, or interests are a few ways to establish rapport.

Assessment

The interview should be conducted in a conversational style using layman's terms. Start the interview by asking questions that are less personal and save more personal questions for later in the interview when more trust has been built. Ask open-ended questions that allow the client the opportunity to tell his story. When the patient is speaking, actively listen to what is being said. Guided questions can be used to get more specific information or to redirect the interview.

Do not use leading questions, as the accuracy of the response is questionable. Closed questions requiring a quick "yes" or "no" response have their place but should be used sparingly. "Yes" responses most likely will require further information from the client. (You will learn more about all of these types of questions in Part 9: Communication.)

Ending

During the interview, analyze the assessment findings to identify areas that would benefit from case management intervention. Close the interview by providing a summary of the information obtained, focusing on the needs and barriers identified. This information can be used to collaborate with the client on goals. Let the client know of any follow-up action you will be taking, including anything they may receive in the mail, any action they should take, and when he will be contacted next. Provide your contact information for any questions or to provide additional information. Finally, thank them for their time and participation.

Remember, we are constantly assessing our clients with each interaction for changes in their condition, response to interventions, and progress toward achieving goals and outcomes. Although the initial assessment is the most comprehensive, the follow-up assessments are also important.

Deep Dive into Assessment Components

Medication Therapy Management and Reconciliation

A CM will rarely have a client who is not taking any medications. It is more likely that clients are taking multiple medications, for multiple conditions, prescribed by multiple providers. It is important to review all prescribed medications, as well as OTC medications and supplements the client is taking. "The best medication reconciliation requires a complete understanding of what the patient was prescribed and what medications the patient is actually taking" (The Joint Commission, 2020).

As defined by The Joint Commission, medication reconciliation is:

> a process of comparing the medications a patient is taking (or should be taking) with newly ordered medications. The comparison addresses duplications, omissions, and interactions, and the need to continue current medications. The types of information that clinicians use to reconcile medications include (among others) medication name, dose, frequency, route, and purpose. (2020)

The Joint Commission goes on to state how medication reconciliation should be performed:

> Obtain and/or update information on the medications the patient is currently taking. This information is documented in a list or other format that is useful to those who manage medications.

> Note 1: The organization obtains the patient's medication information at the beginning of an episode of care. The information is updated when the patient's medications change.

> Note 2: Current medications include those taken at scheduled times and those taken on an as-needed basis.

> Note 3: It is often difficult to obtain complete information on current medications from the patient. A good faith effort to obtain this information from the patient and/or other sources will be considered as meeting the intent. (*National Patient Safety Goals Effective January 2018; Ambulatory Health Care Accreditation Program*, 2018)

URAC, a case management accreditation organization, has additional requirements for medication reconciliation requiring it after discharge home from an inpatient or outpatient facility. It is important to know the accreditation body or bodies that guide the institution you work for or fall under. Your employer will have policies and procedures in place adhering to the guidelines of the accreditation body, and your documentation must show that you are adhering to them.

Assess the client's understanding of why he is prescribed each medication and how to take them properly. Additionally, identify the client's adherence to taking the medications as ordered. If nonadherence is identified, it is important to investigate the reason. Does the client forget to take the medication, not understand how to take it properly, or have difficulty obtaining the medication? When the reason for nonadherence is identified, assist the patient with strategies to become adherent and ensure the prescribing doctor is notified.

The goal of medication reconciliation is to prevent unnecessary health complications from not taking needed medications (ex: insulin for diabetics) and to decrease adverse drug events by reducing medication errors, such as omission, duplication, drug interactions, and dosing errors. Most errors occur during patient transitions in care, including changes in setting, level of care, or practitioner.

When should medication reconciliation occur?
- Any time the patient is moved within the hospital, such as from the ICU to the step-down unit
- Upon transfer to another facility
- Upon discharge from any facility
- At each doctor office visit

At a minimum, perform medication reconciliation upon opening the case, after each hospitalization, and after each visit to the doctor's office.

There are times when expert consultation will be needed for medication management. Pharmacists are a great resource for consultation regarding any medication questions or concerns. If you do not have access to a pharmacist in your organization, contact the patient's pharmacy.

Depression Screening

Most organizations have policies and procedures in place to screen for depression as part of the initial assessment and on a regular basis. This usually includes the assessment tool(s) used during this screening. There are also depression screening tools available online. We will take a quick look at one of the most common tools used today, called the Patient Health Questionnaire.

The Patient Health Questionnaire comes in two parts, part 1 is the Patient Health Questionnaire-2 (PHQ-2) and it pre-screens for depression by asking two questions. *How often over the last two weeks have you (1) Had little interest or pleasure in doing things? and (2) Felt down, depressed or hopeless?*

Clients who pre-screen positive for depression should be evaluated further with the Patient Health Questionnaire-9 (PHQ-9), which is the most common screening tool used to identify depression. It asks the patient to rate the frequency of nine problems occurring over the previous two weeks on a scale ranging from 0 (not at all) to 3 (nearly every day). The first two questions of the PHQ-9 are the same as the PHQ-2. (*Administering the patient health questionnaires 2 and 9 (PHQ 2 and 9) in integrated care settings*, 2018).

Here is a link to an online PHQ-9 calculator: https://www.mdcalc.com/phq-9-patient-health-questionnaire-9

Health Literacy Assessment

Health literacy is not simply the ability to read. Health literacy is the degree to which individuals can find, understand, and use information and services to inform health-related decisions and actions for themselves and others (*Health Literacy in Healthy People 2030 | health.gov*, 2020). It requires a complex set of reading, listening, analytical, and decision-making skills, as well as the ability to apply these skills to health situations.

In addition to basic literacy skills, health literacy requires knowledge of health topics, such as how the body works and the causes of disease. This is the foundation needed to understand treatment options and informed consent documents. Health literacy also requires numeracy skills, such as calculating insulin dosage, measuring medication, understanding nutrition labels, and interpreting lab results. Even successful and well-educated people may have low health literacy abilities.

The National Assessment of Adult Literacy measures the health literacy of adults living in the United States using four basic performance levels: Proficient, Intermediate, Basic, and Below Basic. Only 12% of the population was found to have a proficient health literacy level (*America's health literacy: Why we need accessible health information*, 2008). This means that nearly 9 out of 10 adults in the United States are not proficient in understanding health-related information.

With the knowledge that the vast majority of Americans are not proficient in health literacy, CMs can ask their clients better questions. Instead of asking, "Do you understand your discharge instructions?", it is more appropriate to ask specific questions about how they are taking their medications, when they are following up with their doctor, and which signs and symptoms to report. Use common language, not medical terms, when speaking with patients.

Low health literacy has been linked to higher rates of hospitalization, increased usage of emergency departments, less frequent use of preventive services, and a greater likelihood of taking medicines incorrectly. People with limited health literacy are also more likely to have chronic conditions and are less able to manage them effectively. All of these outcomes are associated with higher healthcare costs (National Library of Medicine, 2010).

Those at highest risk for low health literacy are:
- Older adults
- Racial and ethnic minorities
- Those having less than a high school degree or GED
- Individuals whose income is at or below the poverty level
- Non-native speakers of English (Rikard et al., 2016)

Signs of low health literacy include deferring questions about their health history to a family member, stating that a family member handles their medications, frequent hospitalizations or emergency room visits, misuse of medications, and not being able to verbalize the plan of care.

Use single question assessments to assess health literacy, such as:
- How often do you have someone help you read hospital materials?
- How confident are you in filling out medical forms by yourself?
- How often do you need to have someone help you when you read instructions, pamphlets, or other written material from your doctor or pharmacy?

There are also formal health literacy instruments. The most widely used are:

Rapid Estimate of Adult Literacy in Medicine (REALM) – Assesses the ability of adult patients to read common medical words and lay terms for illnesses and body parts. The examiner scores the patient on the number of words pronounced correctly, but no attempt is made to determine if the patient actually understands the meaning of the word. This assessment is only available in English. View the assessment here: https://www.ahrq.gov/sites/default/files/wysiwyg/professionals/quality-patient-safety/quality-resources/tools/literacy/realm.pdf

The Newest Vital Sign – A tool that tests literacy skills for both numbers and words. It is available in English and Spanish. It is designed to assess a patient's health literacy skills quickly and simply, taking only three minutes to administer. The patient is given a specially designed ice cream nutrition label to review and is asked a series of questions about it. Based on the number of correct answers, healthcare providers assess the patient's health literacy level.

Test of Functional Health Literacy Assessment (TOFHLA) – A more complex assessment that takes 20 minutes or more to administer and consists of two parts, each with different types of questions.

The first part consists of 17 multiple choice questions that test a patient's ability to interpret numbers and documents. The second part assesses reading comprehension by asking patients to read three passages of text in which a blank line replaces keywords. The patient chooses the word that makes the most sense from a word bank. A shorter version of the test is available and is known as the S-TOFHLA. It can be completed in about 12 minutes and contains four multiple-choice questions and two reading passages. Both the TOFHLA and the S-TOFHLA are available in English and Spanish.

Activities of Daily Living (ADLs)

The ADLs and the more advanced instrumental activities of daily living (IADLs) are assessment tools that evaluate areas of essential function for self-care and independence.

ADLs measure the level of independence on performing six basic activities:
- Bathing
- Dressing
- Toileting/continence
- Transferring
- Hygiene/grooming
- Feeding

The IADLs tool assesses the ability to perform eight independent living skills that are more complex than the basic ADLs assessment. These include:

- Shopping
- Using the telephone
- Paying bills/budgeting
- Food preparation
- Housekeeping
- Laundry
- Using transportation
- Handling medications

Substance Use, Abuse, and Addiction

It's imperative to assess for substance abuse or addiction, because it may complicate the diagnosis and/or treatment of medical conditions. Most patients will not readily admit that they have an addiction problem. The CAGE tool is available for screening for substance abuse. It consists of four questions:

- "Have you ever felt you should **C**ut down on drinking/drug use?"
- "Have people **A**nnoyed you by criticizing your drinking/drug use?"
- "Have you ever felt **G**uilty about your drinking/drug use?"
- "Have you ever taken a drink/used drugs in the morning to steady your nerves or get rid of a hangover (**E**ye-opener)?"

Answering yes to two of the questions provides a strong indication of substance abuse. Answering yes to three of the questions confirms the likelihood of substance abuse or dependency.

Part 2: The Case Management Process

Chapter 8

Planning

The objective of the planning phase is to develop an individualized case management plan of care, including goals and interventions, to address the needs and opportunities identified during the initial assessment or at any other time while the client is receiving case management services. This should be completed with input from the client and/or caregiver, providers, and/or an interdisciplinary care team.

Interdisciplinary Care Team (ICT)

An interdisciplinary care team (sometimes referred to as the interdisciplinary team, IDT, interdisciplinary group, IDG, or another term) is a group of healthcare professionals from various professional disciplines who collaborate to manage the physical, psychological, and spiritual needs of the client. When multiple providers, agencies, services, and/or individuals are involved in the provision of care, coordination will be necessary to ensure all needs are met at the appropriate setting, in a timely manner, without duplication of services. This coordination is the responsibility of the CM but requires the involvement and cooperation of others.

In some settings, such as hospice, acute inpatient rehabilitation, long term acute care hospitals (LTACH), and some acute hospitals, the interdisciplinary care team meeting (ICT Meeting) is a formal process done regularly.

Members of the ICT may include:

- Physicians and other primary care providers (PA, NP)
- Nurses
- Case managers
- Social workers
- Physical therapists
- Occupational therapists
- Speech therapists
- Chaplains
- Dieticians
- Pharmacists
- The patient and the patient's family whenever possible

In instances where collaboration, negotiation, and/or problem-solving are needed but ICT meetings are not scheduled, the CM can plan a case conference, inviting providers, family members, and any other members of the IDT. This meeting allows the client's needs to be presented and the team members to collaborate on the best ways to meet those needs.

Both the ICT meeting and the case conference start by reminding everyone why they are there: to develop a plan of care that best meets the needs and goals of the client. Each member of the team introduces themselves and their role in relation to the client. This is especially important if the team is coming together for the first time. Even in an established team, introductions remind everyone of the values each member brings. Each person is to be given an equal opportunity for input and should be asked for their input if it is not volunteered.

Next, the client's case is reviewed, including a brief history, any updates since previous meetings, issues or problems that need to be addressed, and the client's strengths and resources available to him. The remainder of the session involves collaboration on the development of a plan of care or updating the plan of care. Decisions are reached regarding what needs to be done and who is responsible for each task. Creative solutions often result from these types of meetings.

Developing the Case Management Plan of Care

An individualized case management plan of care is developed with input from the client and stakeholders. Stakeholders are those with an interest or concern in the client and may include, but are not limited to, the family, caregiver, primary care physician, specialist(s), hospital or other acute care settings, payer source, and/or any other person or organization with a vested interest in the health of the client. This plan of care should be individualized to the client and recognize the client's desires and preferences as well as be consistent with evidence-based practice when applicable.

The development of a Case Management Plan of Care begins by analyzing all of the information gathered during the assessment phase. The needs and opportunities identified are presented to the client. The CM then helps the client discover goals they will work on together. Interventions are planned to help the client reach his goals.

Long-term goals and short-term goals should be developed and prioritized, and interventions should be planned. Long-term goals are usually those that will take three to six months or longer to reach and can include the client's motivation. For example, a stroke patient's goal may be to walk his daughter down the aisle at her wedding in six months. To accomplish this, he must be able to walk 250 feet with standby assistance.

The short-term goals are goals that, when met, will lead to accomplishing the long-term goal(s), and therefore are directly related to the long-term goals. For our stroke patient mentioned above, his first short-term goal may be to maintain or increase his tolerance so he is able to participate in rehabilitation three hours a day to qualify for inpatient rehabilitation.

The interventions are the treatments, resources, services, and education needed to meet the client's goals. Interventions should apply evidence-based standards and care guidelines when applicable. For our example patient, the interventions the CM and ICT utilize may include educating the client on the importance of tolerating and participating in three hours of therapy a day to reach his goal of walking his daughter down the aisle, bedside physical therapy, and a nutritional plan to give him the required energy and protein.

The acronym SMART is used to identify the attributes of effective goals.
- **S**pecific
- **M**easurable
- **A**chievable
- **R**elevant/Realistic
- **T**ime-based

In addition to being SMART, goals also need to include action words and are individualized to the client.

It is important to note that the outcomes or goals may or may not be clinical. In the example of our stroke patient, the long-term goal is to walk his daughter down the aisle at her wedding in six months. While this long-term goal is not clinical, some of the short-term goals necessary to reach this long-term goal are clinical.

Client participation does not stop with the development of the goals. Clients should also be informed decision-makers in the planning of the interventions. In the example above, the client may have the option of discharging from the acute care hospital to home with home health, or an acute inpatient rehabilitation facility followed by outpatient therapy. There may also be durable medical equipment (DME) needs. The client should be given information on the options available to him, the pros and cons of each, and have assistance in making the best choice to increase the likelihood of reaching his goals. In addition, he should be given choices and input as to the facilities and providers he will use.

Documentation

Just like working in any other area of nursing, if it wasn't documented, it wasn't done. The goals agreed upon are documented in the client's record and reviewed with appropriate stakeholders, documenting their agreement. Accrediting bodies look for this documentation when performing audits. For this reason, it is important to document properly according to your institution's policy. The client record should include documentation of:

- Analysis of the assessment findings supporting the individualized case management plan of care
- The collaboration and communication between team members in developing the plan of care
- Client (or family) participation in the development of the case management plan of care
- Client agreement of the plan of care including goals, expected outcomes, and interventions
- That the client was given the information and resources necessary to make informed decisions
- Any changes or additions to the case management plan of care

The planning phase is completed after services, treatments, and resources needed are identified and authorizations are obtained from the payer. Just like the assessment phase, this planning phase may be revisited as needed.

Case In Point

This case in point focuses on the ICT Meeting for Mr. Carson, a 75-year-old hospice patient with terminal lung cancer. The case manager, hospice aid, physician, hospice chaplain, social worker, dietitian, pharmacist, physical therapist, and Mr. Carson's daughter, Shelly, are present for the meeting.

After introductions are complete, the CM reviews Mr. Carson's case. He was newly admitted to hospice and the entire team has not had a chance to visit Mr. Carson.

The CM explains he was diagnosed with stage 4 lung cancer seven months ago. He underwent chemo and radiation and initially did well, but recently began having issues with anorexia, weight loss, shortness of breath (SOB), and pain. After discussing his options with his physician, the decision was made to begin hospice care.

Mr. Carson lives alone. His daughter lives nearby and checks on him frequently but works full time. She has two teenage children who also check on him.

Recently, he has not been eating the meals prepared for him by his daughter. He eats a few bites and states that is all he can eat. His daughter states she is also concerned that he is unable to properly perform his ADLs due to fatigue. In addition, she is concerned that he lives alone.

He has been rating his pain at 7 consistently, despite the pain medications he is currently on. He is also complaining of increased SOB with minimal exertion. These symptoms, along with his weakness, have resulted in a recent fall.

During his initial assessment, Mr. Carson self-identified as a non-practicing Catholic. He verbalized that he would like to speak to a priest.

Mr. Carson's good support system has been identified as a strength. In addition to his immediate family, there are several nieces and nephews in the area who are willing to assist in his care.

The first issue the team addresses is that Mr. Carson lives alone, as this will impact many of the other issues. His daughter states she would like her father to move in with her and he agreed, but they do not have a first-floor bedroom and bath. This will be extra challenging because he has difficulty using the stairs. The CM states a hospital bed and bedside commode can be obtained. The daughter states that this would work, as they could use the dining room as his bedroom. She is still concerned that he will be home alone for extended periods of time. She agrees to hold a family meeting to schedule drop in's from extended family members throughout the day.

A home health aide will come to her house daily, Monday through Friday, to assist Mr. Carson with his ADLs. This will also provide one hour of supervision for him daily.

Next, his pain is addressed. The pharmacist and physician collaborate on medication changes they believe will alleviate the pain as well as improve his SOB.

The daughter is educated that difficulties with nutrition are common and that the patient should not be forced or pressured to eat. Suggestions are given by the dietitian for high-calorie, easily tolerated foods. She also agrees to meet with him to discuss his preferences.

PT schedules a visit to assess Mr. Carson concerning his recent fall.

The clergy agrees to visit Mr. Carson and if he desires, will contact a local priest and arrange a visit.

With everyone in agreement with the plan of care, the meeting is concluded with an agreement to follow up with another meeting in two weeks.

Chapter 9

Implementation and Coordination of the Case Management Plan of Care

The case management plan of care is proactively carried out during the implementation phase, also called care coordination. The interventions planned in the previous phase are executed, coordinated, and secured. The CM facilitates the coordination of care, transitions of care, services, resources, and health education specified in the planned interventions and acts as a liaison between the client, caregivers, providers, and payer.

To best accomplish this, it is important to understand the role and responsibility of the case manager in relation to that of others involved in providing care and services to the client. This will vary depending on the practice setting the CM is working in. When there is more than one CM involved with the client, it is best if they collaborate early on to determine who is accountable for what actions or goals.

Collaboration with all members of the multidisciplinary healthcare team, community resources, as well as the client and caregiver, is extremely important during planning, coordination, and implementation to facilitate the client's timely receipt of appropriate services. The CM must have excellent communication and organizational skills to effectively collaborate with others and to coordinate care to achieve the goals and outcomes desired.

Special strategies and techniques, such as negotiation techniques and motivational interviewing, are often used to facilitate the achievement of client goals and outcomes. It's important for the CM to have cooperative relationships with all team members involved as she will be the "hub of the wheel," responsible for making sure everything takes place smoothly.

It is not enough to just arrange for the executions of the interventions. It is important to follow up and verify everything is progressing as planned. During transitions of care, successful intervention by the CM will result in the safe transfer of clients to the most appropriate care setting or healthcare provider in a timely manner, and ensure all needed care, services, equipment, medications, and/or treatments are received.

Documentation

All interventions, communications, and education are to be documented in the client record. This documentation should reflect the collaborative communication between the CM, client, and other healthcare team members. It should also demonstrate that the client's needs and preferences were used to guide the facilitation and coordination of services.

Chapter 10

Monitoring and Evaluation

The CM regularly conducts follow-up assessments and continues to gather information from the patient, caregiver, and other relevant sources. This information is evaluated to determine the client's response to the current case management plan and to establish the progress toward the desired outcomes or goals. Modifications are made to the plan as needed, and ongoing follow-ups determine the effectiveness of the modifications.

During these follow-up assessments the CM may monitor for:
- Changes in the client's condition
- Response or lack of response to the case management interventions
- Understanding of teaching provided
- Client satisfaction or request for changes
- Smooth transitions in a care setting or among providers
- Client adherence
- Barriers to care

When necessary, the case management plan of care is revisited and revised based on any new findings. Again, this is done in collaboration with the client, family, caregiver, providers, and/or other pertinent stakeholders.

This is a perfect example of the non-sequential nature of the case management process. We are revisiting the assessment phase while following up to monitor the client and their progress toward reaching the desired goals and outcomes. Although this assessment is more targeted than the comprehensive initial assessment, it is an assessment nonetheless.

Any issues identified with the client's progress toward the outcomes and goals set, or new needs or opportunities that are identified, will lead us back through the planning, implementation, and monitoring phase for those new issues. This will most likely be done concurrently while continuing in the monitoring and evaluation phase for other issues.

Documentation

During this phase it is important to document:

- Follow-up assessment findings
- Client's response to interventions
- Ongoing collaboration with the client, family, caregiver, providers, and/or other pertinent stakeholders
- The plan of care continues to be reviewed
- Any changes or revisions to the case management plan of care

Chapter 11

Closure of Case Management Services

The final step of the case management process is the closure of the client-case manager relationship and engagement in case management services. Each case management program will have its own policies and procedures that must be followed to appropriately close the case. We will look at some universal guidelines to follow based on best practice and CMSA's Standards of Practice.

Ideally, closure to case management services should be mutually agreed upon and occur when the client has met the desired goals and outcomes. Other reasons for closure or termination of case management services may include:

- The client attainment of the highest level of functioning and/or recovery, even if desired goals/outcomes have not been met
- Reaching the maximum benefit from case management services
- Change in the client's healthcare setting, which necessitates the transition of care to another healthcare provider/CM
- The needs and/or desires of the client have changed
- Ongoing client non-compliance, non-adherence, and/or disengagement to the case management plan of care
- Lack of progress toward goals
- Inability to contact the client
- The client refuses further case management services
- Death of the client
- The employer or purchaser of case management services requests the closure of case management

- The client no longer meets the program requirements
- Loss of eligibility for the service before reaching the desired outcomes

It is important to note that when any provider, including a CM, terminates services against the wishes of a client and/or fails to give the client proper notice about the termination of service, especially when leaving the client with unmet needs, it can be considered client abandonment. Client abandonment can result in malpractice claims. For this reason, it is important to strictly follow the case management program's policies and procedures for closing clients to case management services.

It is always best to clearly communicate the expected duration of case management services, and the criteria for continuation in the program from the beginning of the relationship with the client. This conversation can then be revisited as discharge approaches, facilitating the transition out of case management. The purpose and setting of the case management program will often be a major factor in the duration of services. When there is no predetermined date or event for ending services, the CM will need to regularly review whether the case warrants the continuation of the case management relationship with the client.

As closure to case management gets closer, the CM will want to decrease the client's dependence on the CM while fostering independence and self-advocacy. They will also want to gradually decrease the amount of contact with the client as the client functions more independently. These strategies help successfully transition the client out of case management.

Prior to or at discharge, the client should be educated about services and funding resources the CM has put into place, including contact information for any questions, concerns, or future needs. If the client is to be transferred to another facility or provider, a transition of care handover is to be completed and delivered to the providers at the next level of care. This should be done with permission from the client and include information relevant to the continuity of the case management plan of care to optimize client care outcomes.

The work setting of the CM will determine the actual process taken to discharge a client. Ideally, the client is notified verbally and in writing of the closure to case management services. Also, notify the client that they may be asked to complete a patient satisfaction survey regarding the case management services they received.

Documentation

Documentation related to discharge from case management services should include when appropriate:

- Reason for closure
- Client appropriateness for closure
- Client agreement for closure
- Lack of client agreement for closure and supporting documentation to close despite this disagreement
- Client education received on how to follow up regarding services, resources, or funding set up by the CM after the case is closed
- Documentation of the completed transition of care handover to providers at the next level of care, including client permission to disclose this information
- Notice of the closure was communicated to the client (including the form of communication written/verbal)

References

Chapter 5

Case management philosophy and guiding principles | CCMC's case management body of knowledge (CMBOK). (n.d.). Cmbodyofknowledge.com; Commission for Case Management Certification. Retrieved June 25, 2021, from https://cmbodyofknowledge.com/content/case-management-philosophy-and-guiding-principles

Chapter 6

Case Management Society of America. (2016). *Standards of Practice for Case Management* (p. 27). Case Management Society of America.

Chapter 7

Administering the patient health questionnaires 2 and 9 (PHQ 2 and 9) in integrated care settings. (2018, August). www.health.ny.gov; New York State Department of Health. https://www.health.ny.gov/health_care/medicaid/redesign/dsrip/2016-07-01_phq_2_and_9_clean.htm

America's health literacy: Why we need accessible health information. (2008). In *AHRQ* (pp. 1-7). America's health literacy: Why we need accessible health information. https://www.ahrq.gov/sites/default/files/wysiwyg/health-literacy/dhhs-2008-issue-brief.pdf

Health Literacy in Healthy People 2030 | health.gov. (2020, December 3). Health.gov; Office of Disease Prevention and Health Promotion. https://health.gov/our-work/national-health-initiatives/healthy-people/healthy-people-2030/health-literacy-healthy-people-2030

National Library of Medicine. (2010). *Health literacy | NNLM*. Nnlm.gov. https://old.nnlm.gov/initiatives/topics/health-literacy

National Patient Safety Goals Effective January 2018; Ambulatory Health Care Accreditation Program. (2018, January). Jointcommission.org; The Joint Commission. https://www.jointcommission.org/assets/1/6/NPSG_Chapter_AHC_Jan2018.pdf [The 2018 National Patient Safety goals document is no longer available on the Jointcommission.org website; for the National Patient Safety goals effective Jan. 1, 2022, see https://www.jointcommission.org/-/media/tjc/documents/standards/national-patient-safety-goals/2022/npsg_chapter_ahc_jan2022.pdf]

Rikard, R. V., Thompson, M. S., McKinney, J., & Beauchamp, A. (2016). Examining health literacy disparities in the United States: a third look at the national assessment of adult literacy (NAAL). *BMC Public Health, 16*(1). https://doi.org/10.1186/s12889-016-3621-9

The Joint Commission. (2020). National Patient Safety Goals Effective July 2020 for the Ambulatory Health Care Program. In *JointCommsission.org* (p. 4). https://www.jointcommission.org/-/media/tjc/documents/standards/national-patient-safety-goals/2020/npsg_chapter_ahc_jul2020.pdf

Part 3: Ethical, Legal, and Practice Standards

Outcomes

Readers will be able to:

- Identify the case management practice standards
- Identify circumstances that may cause an ethical situation
- Explain the difference between an ethical situation and an ethical dilemma
- Describe the steps to take when faced with an ethical situation
- Explain privacy and confidentiality related to case management
- Identify steps that can be taken to decrease the likelihood of a malpractice suit
- List the criteria that must be met for consent to be informed consent
- Identify important case management legal and regulatory requirements
- Apply healthcare and disability-related legislation to case management

Introduction

The professional CM is a licensed professional who is obligated to work within ethical, legal, and practice standards as required by their license, governing bodies, and accrediting organizations. They have the important role of protecting the rights, dignity, and public interests of their clients. To successfully accomplish these, CMs must understand the standards to which they are held and the legislative mandates impacting the clients' rights, as well as that of their own practice.

There are entire books written on the subject of ethics, and we will not go into a deep dive on the subject. We will instead give you an overview of how the subject relates to case management, as well as the ethical tenets professional case management was built on to provide a better understanding of the practice and standards.

Part 3: Ethical, Legal, and Practice Standards

Chapter 12

Standards of Practice

CMs are held to numerous sets of standards, including:

- Professional standards related to their license

- State practice acts

- Case Management Society of America's Standards of Practice for Case Management

In addition, certified CMs are held to additional standards as per their certifying body.

CMSA's Standards of Practice apply to all CMs and are not limited to members of CMSA. For this reason, it is essential for all CMs to know and understand these standards. These standards will be referenced throughout this book and many of the topics addressed will be covered in greater detail. For now, let's review the standards of practice.

Please note that at the time of this writing, CMSA is currently in the process of updating the 2016 Standards of Practice. At the time of this writing, the 2016 Standards of Practice are the most current. Please contact CMSA for more information on the update.

The following is an excerpt from the CMSA Standards of Practice for Case Management. The full standards are available on their website at: www.cmsa.org

III. Definition of Case Management

The basic concept of case management involves the timely coordination of quality services to address a client's specific needs in a cost-effective and safe manner in order to promote optimal outcomes. This can occur in a single health care setting or during the client's transitions of care throughout the care continuum. The professional case manager serves as an important facilitator among the client, family or family caregiver, the interprofessional health care team, the payer, and the community.

As demonstrated in the section on the Evolution of the Standards of Case Management, the definition of case management has evolved over a period of time; it reflects the vibrant and dynamic progression of the standards of practice.

Following more than a year of study and discussion with members of the national Case Management Task Force, the CMSA's Board of Directors approved a definition of case management in 1993.

Since that time, the CMSA Board of directors has repeatedly reviewed and analyzed the definition of case management to ensure its continued application in the dynamic health environment. The definition was modified in 2002 to reflect the process of case management outlined within the Standards. It was again revisited in 2009 and modified to further align with the practice of case management at the time. The definition was as follows (CMSA, 2009):

Case management is a collaborative process of assessment, planning, facilitation, care coordination, evaluation, and advocacy for options and services to meet an individual's and family's comprehensive health needs through communication and available resources to promote quality cost-effective outcomes.

While one may believe that the 2009 definition of case management remains appropriate today, with the recent focus on client safety, the CMSA Board of Directors has decided to explicitly reference safety in the 2016 definition:

Case Management is a collaborative process of assessment, planning, facilitation, care coordination, evaluation and advocacy for options and services to meet an individual's and family's comprehensive health needs through communication and available resources to promote patient safety, quality of care, and cost effective outcomes.

IV. Philosophy and Guiding Principles

A. Statement of Philosophy

A philosophy is a statement of belief and values that sets forth principles to guide a program, its meaning, its context, and the role of the individual(s) that exist in it. The CMSA's philosophy of case management articulates that:

- The underlying premise of case management is based in the fact that, when an individual reaches the optimum level of wellness and functional capability, everyone benefits: the individual client being served, the client's family or family caregiver, the health care delivery system, the reimbursement source or payer, and other involved parties such as the employer and consumer advocates.

- Professional case management serves as a means for achieving client wellness

Reprinted with permission, the Case Management Society of America, 6301 Ranch Drive, Little Rock, AR 72223, www.cmsa.org.

and autonomy through advocacy, ongoing communication, health education, identification of service resources, and service facilitation.

• Professional case management services are best offered in a climate that allows client's engagement and direct communication among the case manager, the client, the client's family or family caregiver, and appropriate service personnel, in order to optimize health outcomes for all concerned (CMSA, 2009).

The philosophy of case management underscores the recommendation that at-risk individuals, especially those with complex medical, behavioral, and/or psychosocial needs, be evaluated for case management intervention. The key philosophical components of case management address care that is holistic and client-centered, with mutual goals, allowing stewardship of resources for the client and the health care system including the diverse group of stakeholders. Through these efforts, case management focuses simultaneously on achieving optimal health and attaining wellness to the highest level possible for each client.

It is the philosophy of case management that when the provision of health care is effective and efficient, all parties benefit.

Case management, provided as part of a collaborative and interprofessional health care team, serves to identify options and resources which are acceptable to the client and client's family or family caregiver. This then, in turn, increases the potential for effective client's engagement in self-management, adherence to the case management plan of care, and the achievement of successful outcomes.

Case management interventions focus on improving care coordination and reducing the fragmentation of the services the recipients of care often experience especially when multiple health care providers and different care settings are involved. Taken collectively, case management interventions are intended to enhance client safety, well-being, and quality of life. These interventions carefully consider health care costs through the professional case manager's recommendations of cost-effective and efficient alternatives for care. Thus, effective case management directly and positively impacts the health care delivery system especially in realizing the goals of the "Triple Aim" which include improving the health outcomes of individuals and populations, enhancing the experience of health care, and reducing the cost of care.

B. Guiding Principles

Guiding principles are relevant and meaningful concepts that clarify or guide practice. Guiding principles for case management practice provide that professional case managers:

• Use a client-centric, collaborative partnership approach that is responsive to the individual client's culture, preferences, needs, and values.

• Facilitate client's self-determination and self-management through the tenets of advocacy, shared and informed decision-making, counseling, and health education, whenever possible.

• Use a comprehensive, holistic, and compassionate approach to care delivery which integrates a client's medical, behavioral, social, psychological, functional, and other needs.

• Practice cultural and linguistic sensitivity, and maintain current knowledge of diverse populations within their practice demographics.

• Implement evidence-based care guidelines in the care of clients, as available and applicable to the practice setting and/or client population served.

- Promote optimal client safety at the individual, organizational, and community level.

- Promote the integration of behavioral change science and principles throughout the case management process.

- Facilitate awareness of and connections with community supports and resources.

- Foster safe and manageable navigation through the health care system to enhance the client's timely access to services and the achievement of successful outcomes.

- Pursue professional knowledge and practice excellence and maintain competence in case management and health and human service delivery.

- Support systematic approaches to quality management and health outcomes improvement, implementation of practice innovations, and dissemination of knowledge and practice to the health care community.

- Maintain compliance with federal, state, and local rules and regulations, and organizational, accreditation, and certification standards.

- Demonstrate knowledge, skills, and competency in the application of case management standards of practice and relevant codes of ethics and professional conduct.

Case management guiding principles, interventions, and strategies target the achievement of optimal wellness, function, and autonomy for the client and client's family or family caregiver through advocacy, assessment, planning, communication, health education, resource management, care coordination, collaboration, and service facilitation.

The professional case manager applies these principles into practice based on the individualized needs and values of the client to assure, in collaboration with the interprofessional health care team, the provision of safe, appropriate, effective, client-centered, timely, efficient, and equitable care and services.

V. Case Management Practice Settings

Professional case management practice extends to all health care settings across the continuum of health and human services. This may include the payer, provider, government, employer, community, and client's home environment. The practice varies in degrees of complexity, intensity, urgency and comprehensiveness based on the following four factors (Powell and Tahan, 2008; Tahan and Treiger, 2017):

1. The context of the care setting such as wellness and prevention, acute, subacute and rehabilitative, skilled care, or end-of-life.

2. The health conditions and needs of the client population(s) served, and the needs of the client's family or family caregivers.

3. The reimbursement method applied, such as managed care, workers' compensation, Medicare, or Medicaid.

4. The health care professional discipline of the designated case manager such as but not limited to a registered nurse, social worker, physician, rehabilitation counselor, and disability manager.

The following is a representative list of case management practice settings; however, it is not an exhaustive reflection of where professional case managers exist today. Case managers practice in:

- Hospitals and integrated care delivery systems, including acute care, sub-acute care, long-term acute care (LTAC) facilities, skilled nursing facilities (SNFs), and rehabilitation facilities.

- Ambulatory care clinics and community-based organizations, including student or university counseling and health care centers, medical and health homes, primary care practices, and federally qualified health centers.

- Corporations.
- Schools.
- Public health insurance and benefit programs such as Medicare, Medicaid, and state-funded programs.
- Private health insurance programs such as workers' compensation, occupational health, catastrophic and disability management, liability, casualty, automotive, accident and health, long-term care insurance, group health insurance, and managed care organizations.
- Independent and private case management companies.
- Government-sponsored programs such as correctional facilities, military health and Veterans Administration, and public health.
- Provider agencies and community-based facilities such as mental/behavioral health facilities, home health services, ambulatory, and day care facilities.
- Geriatric services, including residential, senior centers, assisted living facilities, and continuing care retirement communities.
- Long-term care services, including home, skilled, custodial, and community based programs.
- End-of-life, hospice, palliative, and respite care programs
- Physician and medical group practices, Patient Centered Medical Home (PCMH), Accountable Care Organizations (ACOs), and Physician Hospital Organizations (PHOs).
- Life care planning programs.
- Population health, wellness and prevention programs, and disease and chronic care management companies.

VI. Professional Case Management Roles and Responsibilities

It is necessary to differentiate between the terms "role," "function," and "activity" before describing the responsibilities of professional case managers. Defining these terms provides a clear and contextual understanding of the roles and responsibilities of case managers in the various practice settings.

A role is a general and abstract term that refers to a set of behaviors and expected consequences that are associated with one's position in a social structure. A function is a grouping or a set of specific tasks or activities within the role. An activity is a discrete action, behavior or task a person performs to address the expectations of the role assumed (Tahan and Campagna, 2010).

A role consists of several functions and each function is described through a list of specific and related activities. These descriptions constitute what is commonly known as a "job description" (Tahan and Campagna, 2010). The roles professional case managers assume may vary based on the same four factors described earlier in the section entitled, Case Management Practice Settings.

The professional case manager performs the primary functions of assessment, planning, facilitation, coordination, monitoring, evaluation, and advocacy. Integral to these functions is collaboration and ongoing communication with the client, client's family or family caregiver, and other health care professionals involved in the client's care. Nationally recognized professional associations and specialty certifying bodies have identified key responsibilities of case managers through expert opinions, practice analyses, and roles and functions research.

It is not the intent of the *Standards of Practice for Case Management* to parallel these key responsibilities. The Standards broadly define major functions involved in the case management process to achieve desired outcomes. The specific roles and responsibilities of professional case managers may vary based on their health discipline background and the environment or care setting they practice in.

Successful care outcomes cannot be achieved without the specialized skills, knowledge, and competencies professional case managers apply throughout the case management process. These include, but are not limited to, motivational interviewing and positive relationship-building; effective written and verbal communication; negotiation and brokerage of services; cost-conscious allocation of resources; knowledge of contractual health insurance or risk arrangements; client activation, empowerment, and engagement; the ability to effect change, perform ongoing evaluation and critical analysis; and the skill to plan, organize, and manage competing priorities effectively.

To facilitate effective and competent performance, the professional case manager should demonstrate knowledge of health insurance and funding sources, health care services, human behavior dynamics, health care delivery and financing systems, community resources, ethical and evidence-based practice, applicable laws and regulations, clinical standards and outcomes, and health information technology and digital media relevant to case management practice. The skills and knowledge base of a professional case manager may be applied to individual clients such as in the hospital setting, or to groups of clients such as in disease, chronic care, or population health management models. Often case managers execute their responsibilities across settings, providers, over time, and beyond the boundaries of a single episode of care. They also employ the use of health and information technology and tools.

The role functions of professional case managers may include, but are not limited to, the following:

- Considering predictive modeling, screening, and other data, where appropriate, in deciding whether a client would benefit from case management services.

- Conducting an assessment of the client's health, physical, functional, behavioral, psychological, and social needs, including health literacy status and deficits, self-management abilities and engagement in taking care of own health, availability of psychosocial support systems including family caregivers, and socioeconomic background. The assessment leads to the development and implementation of a client-specific case management plan of care in collaboration with the client and family or family caregiver, and other essential health care professionals

- Identifying target care goals in collaboration with the client, client's family or family caregiver, and other members of the health care team. Securing client's agreement on the target goals and desired outcomes.

- Planning the care interventions and needed resources with the client, family or family caregiver, the primary care provider, other health care professionals, the payer, and the community-based agents, to maximize the client's health care responses, quality, safety, cost-effective outcomes, and optimal care experience.

- Facilitating communication and coordination among members of the interprofessional health care team, and involving the client in the decision-making process in order to minimize fragmentation in the services provided and prevent the risk for unsafe care and suboptimal outcomes.

- Collaborating with other health care professionals and support service providers across care settings, levels of care, and professional disciplines, with special attention to safe transitions of care.

- Coordinating care interventions, referrals to specialty providers and community-based support services, consults, and resources across involved health providers and care settings.

- Communicating on an ongoing basis with the client, client's family or family caregiver, other involved health care professionals and support service providers, and assuring that all are well-informed and current on the case management plan of care and services.

- Educating the client, the family or family caregiver, and members of the interprofessional health care team about treatment options, community resources, health insurance benefits, psychosocial and financial concerns, and case management services, in order to make timely and informed care-related decisions.

- Counseling and empowering the client to problem-solve by exploring options of care, when available, and alternative plans, when necessary, to achieve desired outcomes.

- Completing indicated notifications for and pre-authorizations of services, medical necessity reviews, and concurrent or retrospective communications, based on payer's requirements and utilization management procedures.

- Ensuring the appropriate allocation, use, and coordination of health care services and resources while striving to improve safety and quality of care, and maintain cost effectiveness on a case-by-case basis.

- Identifying barriers to care and client's engagement in own health; addressing these barriers to prevent suboptimal care outcomes.

- Assisting the client in the safe transitioning of care to the next most appropriate level, setting, and/or provider.

- Striving to promote client self-advocacy, independence, and self-determination, and the provision of client-centered and culturally-appropriate care.

- accommodation(s)

- for both the client and the payer to facilitate positive outcomes for the client, the interprofessional health care team, and the payer. However, when a conflict arises, the needs of the client must be the number one priority.

- Evaluating the value and effectiveness of case management plans of care, resource allocation, and service provision while applying outcomes measures reflective of organizational policies and expectations, accreditation standards, and regulatory requirements.

- Engaging in performance improvement activities with the goal of improving client's access to timely care and services, and enhancing the achievement of target goals and desired outcomes.

VII. Components of the Case Management Process

The case management process is carried out within the ethical and legal realms of a case manager's Scope of practice, using critical thinking and evidence-based knowledge. The overarching themes in the case management process include the activities described below.

Note that the case management process is cyclical and recurrent, rather than linear and unidirectional. For example, key functions of the professional case manager, such as communication, facilitation, coordination, collaboration, and advocacy, occur throughout all the steps of the case management process and in constant contact with the client, client's family or family caregiver, and other members of the interprofessional health care team. Primary steps in the case management process include:

1. Client Identification, Selection and Engagement in Professional Case Management:

- Focus on screening clients identified or referred by other professionals for case management to determine appropriateness for and benefits from services.
- Engagement of the client and family or family caregiver in the process.
- Obtaining consent for case management services as part of the case initiation process.

2. Assessment and Opportunity Identification:

- Assessment begins after screening, identification and engagement in case management. It involves data gathering, analysis, and synthesis of information for the purpose of developing a client-centric case management plan of care.
- Assessment helps establish the client-case manager's relationship and the client's readiness to engage in own health and well-being. It requires the use of effective communication skills such as active listening, meaningful conversation, motivational interviewing, and use of open-ended questions.
- Care needs and opportunities are identified through analysis of the assessment findings and determination of identified needs, barriers, and/or gaps in care.
- Assessment is an ongoing process occurring intermittently, as needed, to determine efficacy of the case management plan of care and client's progress toward achieving target goals.
- Assessment should cover medical, behavioral health, substance use and abuse and social determinants of health.

3. Development of the Case Management Plan of Care:

- The case management plan of care is a structured, dynamic tool used to document the opportunities, interventions, and expected goals, the professional case manager applies during the client's engagement in case management services. It includes:
  - » Identified care needs, barriers and opportunities for collaboration with the client, family and/or family caregiver, and members of the interprofessional care team in order to provide more effective integrated care;
  - » Prioritized goals and/or outcomes to be achieved; and
  - » Interventions or actions needed to reach the goals.
- Client and/or client's family or family caregiver input and participation in the development of the case management plan of care is essential to promote client-centered care and maximize potential for achieving the target goals.

4. Implementation and Coordination of the Case Management Plan of Care:

The case management plan of care is put into action by facilitating the coordination of care, services, resources, and health education specified in the planned interventions.

- Effective care coordination requires ongoing communication and collaboration with the client and/or client's family or family caregiver, as well as the provider and the entire interprofessional health care team.

5. Monitoring and Evaluation of the Case Management Plan of Care:

- Ongoing follow-up with the client, family and/or family caregiver and evaluation of the client's status, goals, and outcomes.

- Monitoring activities include assessing client's progress with planned interventions

- Evaluating if care goals and interventions remain appropriate, relevant, and realistic.

- Determining if any revisions or modifications are needed to the care needs, goals, or interventions specified in the client's case management plan of care

6. Closure of the Professional Case Management Services:

- Bringing mutually-agreed upon closure to the client-case manager relationship and engagement in case management.

- Case closure focuses on discontinuing the professional case management services when the client has attained the highest level of functioning and recovery, the best possible outcomes, or when the needs and desires of the client have changed.

VIII. Standards of Professional Case Management Practice

A. STANDARD: CLIENT SELECTION PROCESS FOR PROFESSIONAL CASE MANAGEMENT SERVICES

The professional case manager should screen clients referred for case management services to identify those who are appropriate for and most likely to benefit from case management services available within a particular practice setting.

How Demonstrated:

- Documentation of consistent use of the client selection process within the organization's policies and procedures.

- Use of screening criteria as appropriate to select a client for inclusion in case management. Examples of screening criteria may include, but are not limited to:
  » Barriers to accessing care and services
  » Advanced age

» Catastrophic or life-altering conditions
» Chronic, complex, or terminal conditions
» Concerns regarding self-management ability and adherence to health regimens
» Developmental disabilities
» End-of-life or palliative care
» History of abuse or neglect
» History of mental illness, substance use, suicide risk, or crisis intervention
» Financial hardships
» Housing and transportation needs
» Lack of adequate social support including family caregiver support
» Low educational levels
» Low health literacy, reading literacy, or numeracy literacy levels
» Impaired functional status and/or cognitive deficits
» Multiple admissions, readmissions, and emergency department (ED) visits
» Multiple providers delivering care and/ or no primary care provider
» Polypharmacy and medication adherence needs
» Poor nutritional status
» Poor pain control
» Presence of actionable gaps in care and services
» Previous home health and durable medical equipment usage
» Results of established predictive modeling analysis and/or health risk screening tools indicative of need for case management
» Risk taking behaviors
» Recognition that a professional case manager may receive pre-screened client referrals from various sources, including (but not limited to) direct referrals from health care professionals and system-generated flags, alerts, or triggers. In

these situations, the case manager should document the referral source and why the client is appropriate for case management services.

B. STANDARD: ASSESSMENT

The professional case manager should complete a thorough individualized client centered assessment that takes into account the unique cultural and linguistic needs of that client including client's family or family caregiver as appropriate.

It is recognized that an assessment:

- is a process, that focuses on evolving client needs identified by the case manager over the duration of the professional relationship and across the transitions of care;
- involves each client and/or the client's family or family caregiver as appropriate, and;
- is inclusive of the medical, cognitive, behavioral, social, and functional domains, as pertinent to the practice setting (Kathol, Perez, & Cohen, 2010) the client uses to access care.

How Demonstrated:

- Documented client assessments using standardized tools, both electronic and written, when appropriate. The assessment may include, but is not limited to the following components:

Medical

- Presenting health status and conditions
- Medical history including use of prescribed or over the counter medications and herbal therapies
- Relevant treatment history
- Prognosis
- Nutritional status

Cognitive and Behavioral

- Mental health
  - » History of substance use
  - » Depression risk screening
  - » History of treatment including prescribed or over the counter medications and herbal therapies
- Cognitive functioning
  - » Language and communication preferences, needs, or limitations
- Client strengths and abilities
  - » Self-care and self-management capability
  - » Readiness to change
- Client professional and educational focus
  - » Vocational and/or educational interests
  - » Recreational and leisure pursuits
- Self-Management and Engagement Status
  - » Health literacy
  - » Health activation level
  - » Knowledge of health condition
  - » Knowledge of and adherence to plan of care
  - » Medication management and adherence
  - » Learning and technology capabilities

Social

- Psychosocial status
  - » Family or family caregiver dynamics
  - » Caregiver resources: availability and degree of involvement
  - » Environmental and residential
- Financial circumstances
- Client beliefs, values, needs, and preferences including cultural and spiritual
- Access to care
  - » Health insurance status and availability of health care benefits
  - » Healthcare providers involved in client's care
  - » Barriers to getting care and resources

- Safety concerns and needs
  - » History of neglect, abuse, violence, or trauma
  - » Safety of the living situation
- Advanced directives planning and availability of documentation
- Pertinent legal situations (e.g. custody, marital discord, and immigration status)

Functional

- Client priorities and self-identified care goals
- Functional status
- Transitional or discharge planning needs and services, if applicable
  - » Health care services currently receiving or recently received in the home setting
  - » Skilled nursing, home health aide, durable medical equipment (DME), or other relevant services
  - » Transportation capability and constraints
  - » Follow-up care (e.g., primary care, specialty care, and appointments)
  - » Safety and appropriateness of home or residential environment
- Reassessment of the client's condition, response to the case management plan of care and interventions, and progress toward achieving care goals and target outcomes.
- Documentation of resource utilization and cost management, provider options, and available health and behavioral care benefits.
- Evidence of relevant information and data required for the client's thorough assessment and obtained from multiple sources including, but not limited to:
  - » Client interviews;
  - » Initial and ongoing assessments and care summaries available in the client's health record and across the transitions of care;

- » Family caregivers (as appropriate), physicians, providers, and other involved members of the interprofessional health care team;
- » Past medical records available as appropriate; and
- » Claims and administrative data.

C. STANDARD: CARE NEEDS AND OPPORTUNITIES IDENTIFICATION

The professional case manager should identify the client's care needs or opportunities that would benefit from case management interventions.

How Demonstrated:

- Documented agreement among the client and/or client's family or family caregiver, and other providers and organizations regarding the care needs and opportunities identified.
- Documented identification of opportunities for intervention, such as:
  - » Lack of established, evidenced-based plan of care with specific goals
  - » Over-utilization or under-utilization of services and resources
  - » Use of multiple providers and/or agencies
  - » Lack of integrated care
  - » Use of inappropriate services or level of care
  - » Lack of a primary provider or any provider
  - » Non-adherence to the case management plan of care (e.g. medication adherence) which may be associated with the following:
    - Low reading level
    - Low health literacy and/or numeracy
    - Low health activation levels
    - Language and communication barriers
  - » Lack of education or understanding of:
    - Disease process
    - Current condition(s)

- The medication list
- Substance use and abuse
- Social determinants of health

» Lack of ongoing evaluation of the client's limitations in the following aspects of health condition:
  - Medical
  - Cognitive and Behavioral
  - Social
  - Functional

» Lack of support from the client's family or family caregiver especially when under stress

» Financial barriers to adherence of the case management plan of care

» Determination of patterns of care or behavior that may be associated with increased severity of condition

» Compromised client safety

» Inappropriate discharge or delay from other levels of care

» High cost injuries or illnesses

» Complications related to medical, psychosocial or functional condition or needs
  - Lack of support from the client's family or family caregiver especially when under stress
  - Frequent transitions between care settings or providers
  - Poor or no coordination of care between settings or providers

D. STANDARD: PLANNING

The professional case manager, in collaboration with the client, client's family or family caregiver, and other members of the interprofessional health care team, where appropriate, should identify relevant care goals and interventions to manage the client's identified care needs and opportunities. The case manager should also document these in an individualized case management plan of care.

How Demonstrated:

- Documented relevant, comprehensive information and data using analysis of assessment findings, client and/or client's family or family caregiver interviews, input from the client's interprofessional health care team, and other methods as needed to develop an individualized case management plan of care.

- Documented client and/or client's family or family caregiver participation in the development of the written case management plan of care.

- Documented client agreement with the case management plan of care, including agreement with target goals, expected outcomes, and any changes or additions to the plan.

- Recognized client's needs, preferences, and desired role in decision-making concerning the development of the case management plan of care.

- Validated that the case management plan of care is consistent with evidence-based practice, when such guidelines are available and applicable, and that it continues to meet the client's changing needs and health condition.

- Established measurable goals and outcome indicators expected to be achieved within specified time frames. These measures could include clinical as well as non-clinical domains of outcomes management. For example, access to care, cost-effectiveness of care, safety and quality of care, and client's experience of care.

- Evidence of supplying the client, client's family, or family caregiver with information and resources necessary to make informed decisions.

- Promoted awareness of client care goals, outcomes, resources, and services included in the case management plan of care.

- Adherence to payer expectations with respect to how often to contact and reevaluate the client, redefine long and short term goals, or update the case management plan of care.

E. STANDARD: MONITORING

The professional case manager should employ ongoing assessment with appropriate documentation to measure the client's response to the case management plan of care.

How Demonstrated:

- Documented ongoing collaboration with the client, family or family caregiver, providers, and other pertinent stakeholders, so that the client's response to interventions is reviewed and incorporated into the case management plan of care.

- Awareness of circumstances necessitatin revisions to the case management plan of care, such as changes in the client's condition, lack of response to the case management interventions, change in the client's preferences, transitions across care settings and/o providers, and barriers to care and services.

- Evidence that the plan of care continues to be reviewed and is appropriate, understood, accepted by client and/or client's family or family caregiver, and documented.

- Ongoing collaboration with the client, family or family caregiver, providers, and other pertinent stakeholders regarding any revisions to the plan of care.

F. STANDARD: OUTCOMES

The professional case manager, through a thorough individualized client centered assessment, should maximize the client's health, wellness, safety, physical functioning, adaptation,

health knowledge, coping with chronic illness, engagement, and self-management abilities.

How Demonstrated:

- Created a case management plan of care based on the thorough individualized client-centered assessment.

- Achieved through quality and cost-efficient case management services, client's satisfaction with the experience of care, shared and informed decision-making, and engagement in own health and health care.

- Evaluated the extent to which the goals and target outcomes documented in the case management plan of care have been achieved.

- Demonstrated efficacy, efficiency, quality, safety, and cost-effectiveness of the professional case manager's interventions in achieving the goals documented in the case management plan of care and agreed upon with the client and/or client's family caregiver.

- Measured and reported impact of the case management plan of care.

- Applied evidence-based adherence guidelines, standardized tools and proven care processes. These can be used to measure the client's preference for, and understanding of:

  » The proposed case management plan of care and needed resources;

  » Motivation to change and demonstrate healthy lifestyle behavior; and

  » Importance of availability of engaged client, family or family caregiver.

- Applied evidence-based guidelines relevant to the care of specific client populations.

- Evaluated client and/or client's family or family caregiver experience with case management services.

- Used national performance measures for transitional care and care coordination such as those endorsed by the regulatory, accreditation, and certification agencies, and health-related professional associations to ultimately enhance quality, efficiency and optimal client experience.

G. STANDARD: CLOSURE OF PROFESSIONAL CASE MANAGEMENT SERVICES

The professional case manager should appropriately complete closure of professional case management services based upon established case closure guidelines. The extent of applying these guidelines may differ in various case management practice and/or care settings.

How Demonstrated:

- Achieved care goals and target outcomes, including those self-identified by the client and/or client's family or family caregiver.
- Identified reasons for and appropriateness of closure of case management services, such as:
  - » Reaching maximum benefit from case management services;
  - » Change of health care setting which warrants the transition of the client's care to another health care provider(s) and/or setting;
  - » The employer or purchaser of case management services requests the closure of case management;
  - » Services no longer meet program or benefit eligibility requirements;
  - » Client refuses further case management services;
  - » Determination by the professional case manager that he/she is no longer able to provide appropriate case management services because of situations such as a client's ongoing disengagement in

self-management and unresolved non-adherence to the case management plan of care;
  - » Death of the client;
  - » There is a conflict of interest; and
  - » When a dual relationship raises ethical concerns.

- Evidence of agreement for closure of case management services by the client, family or family caregiver, payer, professional case manager, and/or other appropriate parties.
- Evidence that when a barrier to closure of professional case management services arises, the case manager has discussed the situation with the appropriate stakeholders and has reached agreement on a plan to resolve the barrier.
- Documented reasonable notice for closure of professional case management services and actual closure that is based upon the facts and circumstances of each individual client's case and care outcomes supporting case closure. Evidence should show verbal and/or written notice of case closure to the client and other directly involved healthcare professionals and support service providers.
- Evidence of client education about service and/or funding resources provided by the professional case manager to addressany further needs of the client upon case closure.
- Completed transition of care handover to health care providers at the next level of care, where appropriate, with permission from client, and inclusive of communication of relevant client information and continuity of the case management plan of care to optimize client care outcomes.

H. STANDARD: FACILITATION, COORDINATION, AND COLLABORATION

The professional case manager should facilitate coordination, communication, and collaboration with the client, client's family or family caregiver, involved members of the interprofessional health care team, and other stakeholders, in order to achieve target goals and maximize positive client care outcomes.

How Demonstrated:

- Recognition of the professional case manager's role and practice setting in relation to those of other providers and organizations involved in the provision of care and case management services to the client.

- Developing and sustaining proactive client-centered relationships through open communication with the client, client's family or family caregiver, and other relevant stakeholders, to maximize outcomes and enhance client's safety and optimal care experience.

- Evidence of facilitation, coordination, and collaboration to support the transitions of care, including:

  » Transfers of clients to the most appropriate health care provider or care setting are coordinated in a timely and complete manner.

  » Documentation reflective of the collaborative and transparent communication between the professional case manager and other health care team members, especially during each transition to another level of care within or outside of the client's current setting.

  » Use of the case management plan of care, target goals, and client's needs and preferences to guide the facilitation and coordination of services and collaboration among members of the interprofessional health care team, client and client's family or family caregiver.

- Adherence to client privacy and confidentiality mandates during all aspects of facilitation, coordination, communication, and

collaboration within and outside the client's care setting.

- Use of special techniques and strategies such as motivational interviewing, mediation, and negotiation, to facilitate transparent communication and building of effective relationships.

- Coordination and implementation of the use of problem-solving skills and techniques to reconcile potentially differing points of view.

- Evidence of collaboration that optimizes client outcomes; this may include working with community, local and state resources, primary care providers, members of the interprofessional health care team, the payer, and other relevant stakeholders.

- Evidence of collaborative efforts to maximize adherence to regulatory and accreditation standards within the professional case manager's practice and employment setting.

I. STANDARD: QUALIFICATIONS FOR PROFESSIONAL CASE MANAGERS

The professional case manager should maintain competence in her/his area(s) of practice by having one of the following:

- Current, active and unrestricted licensure or certification in a health or human services discipline that allows the professional to conduct an assessment independently as permitted within the scope of practice of the discipline; or

- In the case of an individual who practices in a state that does not require licensure or certification, the individual must have a baccalaureate or graduate degree in social work or another health or human services field that promotes the physical, psychosocial, and/or vocational well-being of the persons being served. The degree must be from an institution that is fully accredited by a nationally recognized educational accreditation organization, and;

- The individual must have completed a supervised field experience in case management, health or behavioral health as part of the degree requirements.

How Demonstrated:

- Possession of the education, experience, and expertise required for the professional case manager's area(s) of practice.
- Compliance with national, state, and/or local laws and regulations that apply to the jurisdiction(s) and discipline(s) in which the professional case manager practices.
- Maintenance of competence through participation in relevant and ongoing continuing education, certification, academic study, and internship programs.
- Practicing within the professional case manager's area(s) of expertise, making timely and appropriate referrals to, and seeking consultation with, others when needed.

Supervision

The professional case manager acts in a supervisory and/or leadership role of other personnel who are unable to function independently due to limitations of license and/or education.

Due to the variation in academic degrees and other educational requirements, it is recommended that individuals interested in pursuing a professional case management career seek guidance as to the appropriate educational preparation and academic degree necessary to practice case management. These interested individuals may seek the Case Management Society of America, American Nurses Association, or Commission for Case Manager Certification, or other relevant professional organizations for further advice and guidance.

NOTE: Social workers who are prepared at the CMSA Standards of Practice for Case Management 27 Master's in Social Work (MSW) degree level and educated under a program that would preclude them from sitting for licensure (where required) or practice at the clinical level should consult with their state licensing board to determine if additional education and/or practicum hours are required.

J. STANDARD: LEGAL

The professional case manager shall adhere to all applicable federal, state, and local laws and regulations, which have full force and effect of law, governing all aspects of case management practice including, but not limited to, client privacy and confidentiality rights. It is the responsibility of the professional case manager to work within the scope of his/her license and/ or underlying profession.

NOTE: In the event that the professional case manager's employer policies or those of other entities are in conflict with applicable legal requirements, the case manager should understand that the law prevails. In these situations, case managers should seek clarification of questions or concerns from an appropriate and reliable expert resource, such as a legal counsel, compliance officer, or an appropriate government agency.

1. Standard: Confidentiality and Client Privacy

The professional case manager should adhere to federal, state, and local laws, as well as policies and procedures, governing client privacy and confidentiality, and should act in a manner consistent with the client's best interest in all aspects of communication and recordkeeping whether through traditional paper records and/or electronic health records (EHR).

NOTE: Federal law preempts (supersedes) state and local law and provides a minimum mandatory national standard; states may enlarge client rights, but not reduce them. For those who work exclusively on federal enclaves or on tribal lands, any issues of concern should direct them to the licensing authority and/or federal law.

How Demonstrated:

- Demonstration of up-to-date knowledge of, and adherence to, applicable laws and regulations concerning confidentiality, privacy, and protection of the client's medical information.

- Evidence of a good faith effort to obtain the client's written acknowledgement that she/he has received notice of privacy rights and practices.

2. Standard: Consent for Professional Case Management Services

The professional case manager should obtain appropriate and informed consent before the implementation of case management services.

How Demonstrated:

- Evidence that the client and/or client's family or family caregiver have been thoroughly informed with regard to:
  - » Proposed case management process and services relating to the client's health condition(s) and needs;
  - » Possible benefits and costs of such services;
  - » Alternatives to proposed services;
  - » Potential risks and consequences of proposed services and alternatives; and
  - » Client's right to decline the proposed case management services and awareness of potential risks and consequences of such decision.

- Evidence that the information was communicated in a client-sensitive manner, which is intended to permit the client to make voluntary and informed choices.

- Documented informed consent where client consent is a prerequisite to the provision of case management services.

K. ETHICS

The professional case manager should behave and practice ethically, and adhere to the tenets of the code of ethics that underlie her/his professional credentials (e.g., nursing, social work, and rehabilitation counseling).

How Demonstrated:

- Awareness of the five basic ethical principles and how they are applied. These are:
  - » Beneficence (to do good),
  - » Nonmaleficence (to do no harm),
  - » Autonomy (to respect individuals' rights to make their own decisions),
  - » Justice (to treat others fairly), and
  - » Fidelity (to follow-through and to keep promises).

- Recognition that:
  - » A primary obligation is to the clients cared for, with
  - » A secondary obligation is engagement in and maintenance of respectful relationships with coworkers, employers, and other professionals.
  - » Laws, rules, policies, insurance benefits, and regulations are sometimes in conflict with ethical principles. In such situations, the professional case manager is bound to address the conflicts to the best of her/his abilities and/or seek appropriate consultation.
  - » All clients are unique individuals and the professional case manager engages them without regard to gender identity, race or ethnicity, and practice, religious, other cultural preferences, or socioeconomic status.

- Maintained policies that are universally respectful of the integrity and worth of each person.

L. STANDARD: ADVOCACY

The professional case manager should advocate for the client, client's family or family caregiver, at the service delivery, benefits administration, and policy-making levels. The case manager is uniquely positioned as an expert in care coordination and advocacy for health policy change to improve access to quality, safe, and cost-effective services.

How Demonstrated:

- Documentation demonstrating:
  - » Promotion of the client's self-determination, informed and shared decision-making, autonomy, growth, and self-advocacy.
  - » Education of other health care and service providers in recognizing and respecting the needs, strengths, and goals of the client.
  - » Facilitation of client access to necessary and appropriate services while educating the client and family or family caregiver about resource availability within practice settings.
  - » Recognition, prevention, and elimination of disparities in accessing high-quality care and experiencing optimal client health care outcomes, as related to race, ethnicity, national origin, and migration background; sex and marital status; age, religion, and political belief; physical, mental, or cognitive disability; gender identity or gender expression; or other cultural factors.
  - » Advocacy for expansion or establishment of services and for client-centered changes in organizational and governmental policy.
- Ensuring a culture of safety by engagement in quality improvement initiatives in the workplace.
- Encouraging the establishment of client, family and/or family caregiver advisory councils to improve client-centered care standards within the organization.
- Joining relevant professional organizations in call to action campaigns, whenever possible, to improve the quality of care and reduce health disparities.
- Recognition that client advocacy can sometimes conflict with a need to balance cost constraints and limited resources Documentation indicates that the professional case manager has weighed decisions with the intent to uphold client advocacy, whenever possible.

M. STANDARD: CULTURAL COMPETENCY

The professional case manager should maintain awareness of and be responsive to cultural and linguistic diversity of the demographics of her/his work setting and to the specific client and/or caregiver needs.

How Demonstrated:

- Evidence of communicating in an effective, respectful, and sensitive manner, and in accordance with the client's cultural and linguistic context.
- Assessments, goal-setting, and development of a case management plan of care to accommodate each client's cultural and linguistic needs and preference of services.
- Identified appropriate resources to enhance the client's access to care and improve healthcare outcomes. These may include the use of interpreters and health educational materials which apply language and format demonstrative of understanding of the client's cultural and linguistic communication patterns, including but not limited to speech volume, context, tone, kinetics, space, and other similar verbal/non-verbal communication patterns.
  - » Pursuit of professional education to maintain and advance one's level of

cultural competence and effectiveness while working with diverse client populations.

N. STANDARD: RESOURCE MANAGEMENT AND STEWARDSHIP

The professional case manager should integrate factors related to quality, safety, access, and cost-effectiveness in assessing, planning, implementing, monitoring, and evaluating health resources for client care.

How Demonstrated:

- Documented evaluation of safety, effectiveness, cost, and target outcomes when designing a case management plan of care to promote the ongoing care needs of the client.

- Evidence of follow-through on the objectives of the case management plan of care which are based on the ongoing care needs of the client and the competency, knowledge, and skills of the professional case manager.

- Application of evidence-based guidelines and practices, when appropriate, in recommending resource allocation and utilization options.

- Evidence of linking the client and family or family caregiver with cultural and linguistically appropriate resources to meet the needs and goals identified in the case management plan of care.

- Documented communication with the client and family or family caregiver about the length of time for availability of a necessary resource, potential and actual financial responsibility associated with a resource, and the range of outcomes associated with resource utilization.

- Documented communication with the client and other interprofessional health care team members, especially during care transitions or when there is a significant change in the client's situation.

- Evidence of promoting the most effective and efficient use of health care services and financial resources.

- Documentation which reflects that the intensity of case management services rendered corresponds with the needs of the client.

O. STANDARD: PROFESSIONAL RESPONSIBILITIES AND SCHOLARSHIP

The professional case manager should engage in scholarly activities and maintain familiarity with current knowledge, competencies, case management-related research, and evidencesupported care innovations. The professional case manager should also identify best practices in case management and health care service delivery, and apply such in transforming practice, as appropriate.

How Demonstrated:

- Incorporation of current and relevant research findings into one's practice, including policies, procedures, care protocols or guidelines, and workflow processes, and as applicable to the care setting.

- Efficient retrieval and appraisal of research evidence that is pertinent to one's practice and client population served.

- Proficiency in the application of researchrelated and evidence-based practice tools and terminologies.

- Ability to distinguish peer-reviewed materials (e.g., research results, publications) and apply preference to such work in practice, as available and appropriate.

- Accountability and responsibility for own professional development and advancement.

- Participation in ongoing training and/ or educational opportunities (e.g., conferences, webinars, academic programs) to maintain and expand one's skills, knowledge and competencies.

- Participation in research activities which support quantification and definition of valid and reliable outcomes, especially those that demonstrate the value of case management services and their impact on the individual client and population health.

- Identification and evaluation of best practices and innovative case management interventions.

- Leveraging opportunities in the employment setting to conduct innovativeperformance improvement projects and formally report on their results.

- Dissemination, through publication and/ or presentation at conferences, of practice innovations, research findings, evidencebased practices, and quality or performance improvement efforts.

- Membership in professional case management-related associations and involvement in local, regional, or national committees and taskforces.

- Mentoring and coaching of less experienced case managers, other interprofessional health care team members, and providers.

Chapter 13

Case Management Ethics

Many circumstances can cause an ethical situation for the CM, including, but not limited to:

- Duty and obligation to multiple people and organizations (e.g., client/employer, client/provider, client/payer)

- Client advocacy vs. cost saving

- CM's influence on the client

- Client's values conflicting with the CM's values

- Client autonomy vs. client safety

- Client advocacy vs. family's or caregiver's wishes

- Advance directives

- Surrogate decision-making

- Refusal of treatment

With the advances of medical intervention, end-of-life care is full of potential ethical dilemmas, ranging from the use of heroic measures to sustain life to assisted suicide. Other ethical issues at the end-of-life can be related to advance directives, pain control, prolonging life, avoiding prolonged suffering, artificial nutrition and hydration, and forgoing treatment.

Understanding the underlying values and principles of case management is important in resolving ethical situations and dilemmas, whether they are related to end-of-life issues, experimental treatments, refusal of care, or any other reason. Case management values are based on the belief that case management is a means for improving client health, wellness, and autonomy through advocacy, communication, education, identification of service resources, and service facilitation (*Case management philosophy and guiding principles I CCMC's case management body of knowledge (CMBOK)*, n.d.).

The underlying principles of case management are:
- The primary obligation is to the client
- Placing public interest above one's own interest at all times
- Respecting the rights and inherent dignity of all clients
- Maintaining objectivity in relationships with clients
- Engaging in respectful relationships with coworkers, employers, and other professionals
- Acting with integrity in dealing with other professionals to facilitate maximum assistance for the client
- Maintaining a level of competency that ensures each client will receive services appropriate and consistent for the client's conditions and circumstances
- Obeying laws and regulations (Commission for Case Management Certification (CCMC), 2018)

An ethical situation can become an ethical dilemma when there is no "right" answer. To be a true ethical dilemma, three conditions must be present.
1. There is a decision the individual must make.
2. There must be different courses of action to choose from.
3. No matter which course of action is taken, an ethical principle is compromised (Allen, 2018).

When faced with a possible or an actual ethical situation, the CM will reference CMSA's Standards of Practice, Ethics Standard, as well as the Code of Ethics for the professional credential that she holds. For nurses, this would be the ANA Code of Ethics for Nurses with Interpretive Statements. These documents will help guide the CM through many ethical issues.

Help may also be found by reviewing the ethical tenets of case management: beneficence, nonmalfeasance, autonomy, justice, fidelity, and veracity. The ethical principle of beneficence, to do good, directs CMs to promote the interests of their clients above all others. This aligns with the CM's role as a client advocate.

In contrast, the principle of nonmalfeasance instructs us to do no harm. This extends to the healthcare services, interventions, and treatments that CMs recommend. Many treatments have a risk of harm to the patient along with the desired benefit. Educate the client so they can make an informed decision, with full knowledge of the potential harm as well as benefit.

This leads us to the principle of autonomy, the client's right to make his own decisions. While the CM gives the client the information he needs to make an informed decision, she must be careful not to influence the client's decision-making but instead foster the client's independence and self-determination.

Veracity is the act of telling the truth. For a client to make an informed decision, he must have truthful, relevant, and understandable information. Fidelity is following through on one's promises. This can be as simple as the CM doing what she said she would do when she said she would do it. This builds the trust needed to work with the client in an impactful way. And finally, justice means treating others fairly. You can begin to see how all of these tenets are interwoven, and if one is missing it impacts the others.

There will be times when an ethical dilemma is faced that cannot be resolved by referencing these resources. This may occur when a law, regulation, policy, or insurance contract benefit conflicts with an ethical principle, or when either course of action will result in the compromising of an ethical principle. When this occurs CMSA's Standards of Practice state that "the professional case manager is bound to address the conflicts to the best of her/his abilities and/or seek appropriate consultation" (CMSA, 2016).

If the policies and procedures of a CM's employer do not align with the legal requirements, the law supersedes policies. CMSA's Standards of Practice 2016 instructs CMs to obtain clarification of questions or concerns from an appropriate and reliable expert resource, such as a legal counsel, compliance officer, or an appropriate government agency (CMSA, 2016).

Reflect on ethical situations you have encountered in your career. Review the conditions that create an ethical dilemma.

Do any of your situations meet the criteria for an ethical dilemma? How did you handle them? Looking back, how could you have handled the situation better?

Chapter 14

Privacy and Confidentiality

Privacy and confidentiality are such important matters that these subjects are covered in:

- Health Insurance Portability and Accountability Act (HIPAA)
- CMSA's Standards of Practice
- Commission for Case Management Certification Code of Professional Conduct
- URAC and the National Committee for Quality Assurance (NCQA) standards
- Federal, state, and local laws
- Employer policies and procedures

When the patient is a minor it is important to be aware of the age of consent in the state where the minor is, as this will determine who gives the informed consent and who is permitted to receive information.

HIPAA specifically covers protected health information (PHI) released, transferred, or divulged outside of the agency. To release this information authorization for the release of PHI should be in place. According to HIPAA, this authorization must be in plain, understandable language, and contain a detailed description of the information to be released, the purpose of the disclosure, the individual's right to revoke the authorization, and the expiration date of the authorization.

HIPAA compliance is required when using fax, phone, and internet communications. The act covers not only formal records but also personal notes and billing information. The CM's client records kept in any form, including written, recorded, computerized, or stored on another medium, must be maintained in a manner to ensure confidentiality. The safeguards include electronic security of files (such as passwords), the security of work areas, and the destruction of files/information. When destroying these records, it must be done in a manner ensuring the preservation of confidentiality. To meet HIPAA requirements, employers will have policies and procedures in place safeguarding privacy and confidentiality as well as a privacy officer.

Information released to another organization under HIPAA becomes protected under the confidentiality guidelines of the organization receiving the information. HIPAA does not apply to disability, auto, liability, or workers' compensation insurance, although a state may have laws that apply to these. Because HIPAA is a federal law, it supersedes state and local laws. It is important to note that state laws take precedence over HIPAA if they are more strict in protecting the privacy of medical records (U.S. Department of Health and Human Services, 2013).

Practical Application/Best Practice for Case Managers

The CMSA's Standards of Practice, certification bodies such as the Commission for Case Management Certification's Code of Professional Conduct, the American Case Management Association as well as URAC and NCQA standards, deal with privacy and confidentiality directly related to case management. Based on their standards, best practice for case managers includes the following practical applications.

At the beginning of the CM and client relationship, CMs are to inform their clients that although their conversations are confidential, certain information obtained through the relationship may be disclosed to third parties, including payers, service providers, and government authorities. The information shared is limited to what is necessary and relevant. If the case management program has notice of its privacy policy, this should be given to the client and written confirmation of receipt received from the client.

In many organizations, a HIPAA/PHI release will be obtained when opening the case to case management. In some settings, such as inpatient or home care where case management is part of the organization's overall treatment, there is one general release covering all aspects of care, and a separate release for case management is not necessary.

Chapter 15

Legal and Regulatory Requirements

Malpractice

Case managers are at risk for malpractice lawsuits even though they do not provide direct patient care. Patients most frequently file malpractice claims when they feel the provider was discourteous and did not take time to listen or explain the care to them. Thus, it often comes down to the basics of communication. When a client feels the provider has listened, understood, and been respectful, he is unlikely to seek legal action.

A malpractice lawsuit can arise from an act of omission (failure to do something that should be done) or an act of commission (doing something that should not be done). Either of these is a breach of obligation. The plaintiff, the person bringing forth the malpractice claim, has the burden of proving two points: the CM was negligent, and an injury resulted from the negligence. To do so, four legal elements must be proven: (1) a professional duty owed to the patient; (2) breach of such duty; (3) injury caused by the breach; and (4) resulting damages.

A CM can take several steps to reduce the risk of a malpractice lawsuit:
- Use only credentialed healthcare providers
- Offer the patient several choices for providers (document these options)
- Communicate with the patient and address concerns
- Document all communications with the patient and others involved in care and decision-making

- Do not alter records
- Follow employer policies and procedures
- Use written guidelines when available; if deviating from them, document justification
- Document compliance or lack of compliance with the treatment plan
- Be aware of and comply with professional standards and regulations

Informed Consent

Unlike malpractice law, under tort law, a medical professional can be liable if informed consent is not obtained before treating the patient, even if there is no injury or the patient is benefited. For example, if consent is obtained for surgery on the right eye and the surgeon performs surgery on the left eye while the patient is under anesthesia, a medical battery has occurred. The surgeon can be held liable because they touched the patient without the patient's consent (permission was given on the right eye, not the left). A tort is a wrongful act or an infringement of a right. Other torts include negligence, false imprisonment, and assault (Gillingham, 2020).

The following criteria must be met for consent to be informed:
- It must include a discussion of possible side effects, risks, consequences, and benefits of treatment, medication, or procedures; including consequences or risks of stoppage of the service
- The client must have the capacity to make clear, competent decisions
- Consent must be self-determined; it cannot be coerced or pressured by the agency or provider of services
- Information must be clear and easy to understand
- Information must be given verbally and in writing
- The patient must have an opportunity for questions and answers

CMSA's Standards of Practice for Case Management as well as URAC state consent for case management services should be obtained prior to the implementation of case management services. This consent should show information was communicated regarding the case management process and services, possible benefits and costs of such services, alternatives, risks, and consequences of services, client's right to decline case management, and the potential risks and consequences of declining (CMSA, 2016).

As covered in Part 2: The Case Management Process, Chapter 6, CMs need to obtain consent for case management as per the policies of the institution where they are employed. Hospital case management is generally understood to be covered under the consent for treatment signed upon hospitalization.

Some states do not require consent in Workers' Compensation case management, but this is changing. Even if the institution you work for does not require written consent for case management services, it is best practice, and part of CMSA's Standards of Practice, to obtain informed consent for case management services. If there is no written consent available in your case management program, then this can be done verbally and must be documented in the client record.

Interstate Compact for Nursing

Nurse CMs must be licensed in the state where case management is being provided. Telephonic CMs who manage cases across state lines must be licensed in the state where the client is located.

The Nurse Licensure Compact gives nurses the ability to practice nursing across state lines. The nurse must be licensed in his or her state of residency. If the state of residency participates in the compact, he or she can practice in any other compact state.

Negligent Referral

Referral of a patient to a healthcare provider who is known to be unqualified is considered a negligent referral. The CM can be held liable for a negligent referral even if she is unaware the provider is unqualified. A reasonably prudent CM is expected to make sure the referred provider is professionally qualified and without physical or mental impairment that could result in harm to the patient.

CMs can verify the qualifications of providers using their organization's network of preferred providers. These providers undergo a routine screening process to meet the requirements to participate in the network of preferred providers.

Another way to verify the quality of providers is to use Medicare approved providers. Medicare approved providers are healthcare providers like home health agencies, hospitals, nursing homes, or dialysis facilities that have been approved by Medicare. Providers are approved or "certified" by Medicare if they've passed an inspection conducted by a state government agency.

Part 3: Ethical, Legal, and Practice Standards

Chapter 16

Healthcare and Disability-Related Legislation

To protect the rights of your clients, you must know the client's rights. Become familiar with the following healthcare and disability-related legislation to learn about clients' rights.

The Americans with Disabilities Act

The Americans with Disabilities Act (ADA) defines an individual with a disability as a person who: 1) has a physical or mental impairment that substantially limits a major life activity, 2) has a record or history of a substantially limiting impairment, or 3) is regarded or perceived by an employer as having a substantially limiting impairment (U.S. Department of Justice Civil Rights Division Disability Rights Section, 2020).

The ADA also protects qualified individuals with prior drug addiction if they have been rehabilitated. However, the ADA provides that the term "individual with a disability" does not include an individual who is currently engaging in the illegal use of drugs.

Assessments are done on a case-by-case basis to determine if the impairment is protected under ADA. An individual, not his or her disability, is protected under ADA.

The ADA prohibits discrimination against people with disabilities in employment, transportation, public accommodation, communications, and governmental activities (U.S. Department of Justice Civil Rights Division Disability Rights Section, 2020).

Employers with 15 or more employees are prohibited from discriminating against people with disabilities by Title I of the ADA. In general, the employment provisions of the ADA require:

- Equal opportunity in selecting, testing, and hiring qualified applicants with disabilities
- Job accommodation for applicants and workers with disabilities when such accommodations would not impose "undue hardship" on the employer
- Equal opportunity in promotion and benefits

An applicant with a disability, like all other applicants, must be able to meet the employer's requirements for the job, such as education, training, employment experience, skills, or licenses. In addition, an applicant with a disability must be able to perform the "essential functions" of the job, either on his or her own or with the help of "reasonable accommodation."

A job accommodation is a reasonable adjustment to a job or work environment that makes it possible for an individual with a disability to perform job duties. Determining whether to provide accommodations involves considering the required job tasks and the functional limitations of the person doing the job.

An employer does not have to provide an accommodation that will cause "undue hardship," defined as being significantly difficult or expensive for the employer. Accommodations may include specialized equipment (such as speech-to-text software or an elevated desk to fit a wheelchair), facility modifications (wheelchair ramps), and adjustments to work schedules or job duties, as well as a range of other creative solutions. The Job Accommodation Network (JAN) provides free consulting on workplace accommodations.

During the application/interview process, the ADA prohibits asking questions such as:

- Do you have a heart condition?
- Do you have asthma or any other difficulties breathing?
- Do you have a disability that would interfere with your ability to perform the job?
- How many days were you sick last year?
- Have you ever filed for workers' compensation?
- Have you ever been injured on the job?
- Have you ever been treated for mental health problems?
- What prescription drugs are you currently taking?

An employer can ask all of the questions listed above and others that are likely to reveal the existence of a disability after the extension of a job offer as long as the same questions are asked of other applicants offered the same type of job. In other words, an employer cannot ask such questions only to those who have obvious disabilities.

Similarly, an employer may require a medical examination and/or drug screen after making a job offer as long as it requires the same medical examination and/or drug screen of all applicants offered the same type of job. The employer can withdraw the job offer only if it can show that the potential employee is unable to perform the essential functions of the job (with or without reasonable accommodation), or that the applicant poses a significant risk of causing substantial harm to himself or others.

COBRA

In 1986, Congress passed the Consolidated Omnibus Budget Reconciliation Act (COBRA). Under this law, employees and their families who might otherwise lose their health insurance due to job loss, decreased work hours, a transition between jobs, death, divorce, and other life events can choose to keep their insurance. Employers (private sector or state/local government) with 20 or more employees offer COBRA.

If a person elects COBRA coverage, he continues to receive group health benefits from the plan for a limited time. The duration of coverage under COBRA is usually 18 months but can last up to 36 months under certain circumstances. In the event of the death of the employee or legal separation or divorce from the employee, the spouse and dependent children are eligible to receive COBRA coverage for 36 months. If the employee or eligible dependent is qualified to receive COBRA due to termination or reduction of hours, and then becomes disabled on or before day 60 of COBRA, he is eligible for 29 months of coverage.

The eligible person must elect COBRA within 60 days of the plan coverage terminating. After the initial election, the first premium payment must be made within 45 days. After this, payments are due on the first of each month, subject to a 30-day grace period. If payments are not made as stated, coverage may be terminated.

A person receiving COBRA benefits may be required to pay the entire premium (including the portion previously paid by the employer), as well as a 2% fee. Thus, COBRA may cost up to 102% of the plan's premium, putting COBRA financially out of reach for many of the people who qualify for it (Employee Benefits Security Administration; United States Department of Labor, 2018).

Family Medical Leave Act (FMLA)

The Family and Medical Leave Act (FMLA) provides eligible employees up to 12 workweeks of unpaid leave a year for specified family and medical reasons. It requires group health benefits to be maintained during the leave as if the employee continued to work. Employees are also entitled to return to their same or an equivalent job at the end of their FMLA leave.

Eligible employees are those who:
- Work for a covered employer (public agencies, including government and local schools, as well as private sector employees working for companies with 50 or more employees within a 75-mile radius of the worksite)
- Have worked 1,250 hours during the 12 months before the start of the leave
- Have worked for the employer for 12 months

FMLA may be taken for:
- Birth, adoption, or foster care of a child
- Care of a spouse, child, or parent who has a serious health condition
- A serious health condition that makes the employee unable to perform the essential functions of his or her job

FMLA does not have to be taken all at once; it can be taken intermittently—taking leave in blocks of time for a single qualifying reason—or to reduce the employee's daily or weekly work schedule. The employer chooses how to count the year; calendar year, any fixed 12 months, the 12-month period measured forward, or a rolling 12 month period measured backward. This must be uniform for all employees.

The FMLA only requires that employers provide unpaid leave. However, the law permits an employee to elect, or the employer to require, that the employee use accrued paid vacation leave or paid sick or family leave for some or all of the FMLA leave period. An employee must follow the employer's normal leave rules in order to substitute paid leave. When paid leave is used for an FMLA-covered reason, the leave is FMLA-protected. If the leave is unpaid, the employee must continue to pay his portion of the medical insurance that was normally deducted from his paycheck (U.S. Department of Labor, 2009).

Mental Health Parity Acts

Mental Health Parity Act of 1996

The Mental Health Parity Act of 1996 does not mandate mental health benefits be offered in health insurance plans. However, it does require that when this benefit is provided, the lifetime or annual dollar limits on mental health care must be the same as the limits that apply to medical or surgical benefits. Substance abuse and chemical dependency are not covered under this act.

The Paul Wellstone and Pete Domenici Mental Health Parity and Addiction Equity Act of 2008 (MHPAEA)

The Paul Wellstone and Pete Domenici Mental Health Parity and Addiction Equity Act of 2008 (MHPAEA) expanded on the MHPA of 1996. This federal law prevents group health plans and health insurance issuers that provide mental health and substance use disorder (MH/SUD) benefits from imposing less favorable benefit limitations on those benefits than on medical/surgical coverage. This applies to:

- Copays, coinsurance, deductibles, and out-of-pocket maximums
- Limitations on service utilization, such as limits on the number of inpatient days or outpatient visits covered
- Coverage for out-of-network providers

The Wellstone-Domenici Parity Act amended and substantially increased the mental health benefits protection afforded under the federal Mental Health Parity Act of 1996, which only required parity coverage for lifetime and annual dollar limits and did not apply to benefits for substance use disorders (The Mental Health Parity and Addiction Equity Act (MHPAEA) | CMS, 2010).

The Affordable Care Act (ACA)

The Affordable Care Act (ACA) expands the MHPAEA of 2008. As stated previously, the MHPAEA of 2008 does not mandate mental health and addiction benefits be offered in health insurance plans.

The ACA further expands the MHPAEA by requiring the coverage of:

- Behavioral health treatment, such as psychotherapy and counseling
- Mental and behavioral health inpatient services
- Substance use disorder treatment
- Alcohol misuse screening and counseling
- Depression screening
- Tobacco use screening and cessation interventions
- Domestic and interpersonal violence screening and counseling
- Behavioral assessment for children

Summary

The MHPA requires large group health plans to not impose annual or lifetime dollar limits on mental health benefits that are less favorable than any such limits imposed on medical/surgical benefits.

MHPAEA preserves the MHPA protections and adds significant new protections, such as extending the parity requirements to substance use disorders. Although the law requires general equality in the way MH/SUD and medical/surgical benefits are treated with respect to annual and lifetime dollar limits, financial requirements, and treatment limitations, MHPAEA does NOT require large group health plans or health insurance issuers to cover MH/SUD benefits. The law's requirements apply only to large group health plans and health insurance issuers that choose to include MH/SUD benefits in their benefits packages.

However, the Affordable Care Act builds on MHPAEA and requires coverage of mental health and substance use disorder services as one of 10 Essential Health Benefits (EHB) categories in non-grandfathered individual and small group plans.

Pregnancy Discrimination Act of 1978

The Pregnancy Discrimination Act:
- Forbids discrimination based on pregnancy in any aspect of employment, including hiring, firing, pay, job assignments, leave, and health insurance
- Requires health insurance provided by the employer to cover expenses for pregnancy-related conditions on the same basis as costs for other medical conditions
- Ensures employees on leave due to pregnancy-related conditions are treated the same as temporarily disabled employees

Newborns' and Mothers' Health Protection Act of 1996

The Newborns' and Mothers' Health Protection Act requires that health plans and insurance issuers don't restrict a mother's or newborn's benefits for a hospital stay connected to childbirth to less than 48 hours following a vaginal delivery or 96 hours following a delivery by cesarean section. However, the attending provider (who may be a physician or nurse midwife) may decide, after consulting with the mother, to discharge the mother or newborn child earlier. Incentives (either positive or negative) that could encourage an attending provider to give less than the minimum protections under the act as described above are prohibited.

Women's Health and Cancer Rights Act of 1998

The act requires that group health plans providing coverage for mastectomies also cover the following:

- Reconstruction of the breast that was removed by mastectomy
- Surgery and reconstruction of the other breast to make the breasts appear symmetrical
- Breast prostheses
- Complications at all stages of mastectomy, including lymphedema

Affordable Care Act (ACA)

The Affordable Care Act (ACA) has created comprehensive health insurance reforms designed to improve access, affordability, and quality in healthcare. Since its signing on March 23, 2010, the law was gradually phased in over five years and is now in full effect. The following is an overview of the key aspects of the law relevant to case management.

End to pre-existing condition discrimination

Insurance companies can no longer deny coverage or charge more because of a pre-existing condition. They also cannot charge more based on gender. Once insured, the insurance company cannot refuse to cover treatment for pre-existing conditions. The one exception to this is grandfathered individual health insurance policies bought on or before March 23, 2010 (Health insurance rights & protections, 2018).

Keeps young adults covered

Adult children who cannot get coverage through their jobs may remain on their parents' policies until they are 26 years old (Health insurance rights & protections, 2018).

Free preventive care benefits

Insurers are now required to cover many recommended preventive services without additional cost-sharing such as copays or deductibles. Depending on age, these preventive services include:

- Blood pressure screening, diabetes, and cholesterol testing
- Some cancer screenings, including mammograms and colonoscopies
- Counseling on topics such as smoking cessation, weight loss, healthy eating, treating depression, and reducing alcohol use

- Well-baby and well-child visits from birth to age 21
- Routine vaccinations
- Counseling, screening, and vaccines to ensure healthy pregnancies
- Flu and pneumonia shots

It is important to note that grandfathered plans may not provide these preventive benefits for free. Also, the health plan can require the use of network providers to receive these benefits without cost-sharing. If something is found during the well visit, it no longer falls under preventive care and is subject to cost-sharing. Finally, there may still be a fee for the office visit related to these services.

Coverage of essential health benefits

All plans offered in the individual and small group markets must cover a comprehensive package of items and services known as essential health benefits. In addition, states expanding their Medicaid programs must provide these benefits to people newly eligible for Medicaid.

Essential health benefits must include items and services within at least the following 10 categories:

- Ambulatory patient services
- Emergency services
- Hospitalization
- Maternity and newborn care
- Mental health and substance use disorder services, including behavioral health treatment (this includes counseling and psychotherapy)
- Prescription drugs
- Rehabilitative and habilitative services and devices
- Laboratory services
- Preventive and wellness services and chronic disease management
- Pediatric services, including oral and vision care (but adult dental and vision coverage are not essential health benefits) (Find out what Marketplace health insurance plans cover, 2019)

These essential health benefits are subject to deductibles and copays. In addition, self-funded employer plans and grandfathered plans are not required to cover these benefits.

End to dollar limits on care

The ACA bans annual and lifetime dollar limits on most covered health benefits (Health insurance rights & protections, 2018). In the past, people with cancer or other illnesses could lose their insurance coverage when their healthcare expenses reached the dollar limit on their policy. There are some exceptions to this ban on limits—for example, grandfathered individual plans are not required to follow the rules on annual limits—and plans can put an annual dollar limit and a lifetime dollar limit on spending for healthcare services that are not essential health benefits.

Ensuring coverage for individuals participating in clinical trials

Insurers are prohibited from dropping or limiting coverage because an individual chooses to participate in a clinical trial. This applies to all clinical trials that treat cancer or other life-threatening diseases.

Guaranteed right to appeal

Under the ACA, the participant has the right to appeal a health insurance company's decision to deny payment for a claim or to terminate health coverage (Health insurance rights & protections, 2018). The participant will first request an internal appeal. If the insurance company upholds its decision to deny payment or coverage, the law permits the participant to request an external review. In an external review, an independent third party decides whether to uphold or overturn the insurance company's decision.

Expands the Mental Health Parity and Addiction Equity Act (MHPAEA) of 2008

As stated previously, the MHPA does not mandate mental health benefits be offered in health insurance plans. It does require that when this benefit is provided, the lifetime or annual dollar limits on mental health care must be the same as the limits that apply to medical or surgical benefits. Substance abuse and chemical dependency are not covered under the MHPAEA. The ACA further expands the MHPAEA by requiring the coverage of:

- Behavioral health treatment, such as psychotherapy and counseling
- Mental and behavioral health inpatient services
- Substance use disorder treatment
- Alcohol misuse screening and counseling
- Depression screening

- Tobacco use screening and cessation interventions
- Domestic and interpersonal violence screening and counseling
- Behavioral assessment for children (Mental health and substance abuse health coverage options, 2019)

Paying physicians based on value not volume

A provision that took effect in 2015 ties physician Medicare payments to the quality of care they provide. Medicare payments will be modified so physicians who provide higher value care will receive higher payments than those who provide lower-quality care.

Linking payment to quality outcomes

The law established a Hospital Value-Based Purchasing program (HVBP) in traditional Medicare. This program offers financial incentives to hospitals to improve the quality of care. It is based on either: 1) how well they perform on each measure compared to other hospitals, or 2) how much they improved their own performance on each measure compared to their performance during a prior baseline period. Hospital performance is required to be publicly reported, beginning with measures relating to heart attacks, heart failure, pneumonia, surgical care, healthcare-associated infections, and patients' perception of care.

Hospital Readmissions Reduction Program

The ACA authorizes Medicare to reduce payments to acute care hospitals with excess readmissions that are paid under CMS's Inpatient Prospective Payment System (IPPS). Excess readmissions are measured by a ratio, by dividing a hospital's number of "predicted" 30-day readmissions for heart attack, heart failure, pneumonia, hip/knee replacement, and COPD, by the number that would be "expected," based on an average hospital with similar patients. A ratio greater than one indicates excess readmissions.

The ACA also identifies ways to improve the often-fragmented healthcare system, such as the patient-centered medical home and the accountable care organization. Both of these rely on care coordination as a central pillar of their success.

Impact for case management

The ACA provides many incentives to improve quality, coordinate care, and decrease costs—all areas where CMs are well-positioned to take the lead. The impact CMs can have in this new value-driven care world is tremendous. Case management functions, such as assessing, planning, educating, discharge planning, care transitioning, care coordination, and monitoring, are key to meeting the savings benchmarks and quality performance standards outlined in the ACA.

References

Chapter 13

Allen, K. (2018, October 12). *What Is an Ethical Dilemma?* SocialWorker.com. https://www.socialworker.com/feature-articles/ethics-articles/What_Is_an_Ethical_Dilemma%3F/

Case Management Society of America. (2016). *Standards of Practice for Case Management* (pp. 12, 13, 27–28). Case Management Society of America.

Commission for Case Management Certification (CCMC). (2018). Code of professional conduct for case managers with standards, rules, procedures, and penalties. In *CCM Certification* (p. 2). https://ccmcertification.org/sites/default/files/docs/2018/ccmc-18-code-of-conduct_1.pdf

Chapter 14

U.S. Department of Health and Human Services. (2013, July 26). *Summary of the HIPAA privacy rule*. HHS.gov. https://www.hhs.gov/hipaa/for-professionals/privacy/laws-regulations/index.html

Chapter 15

Case Management Society of America. (2016). *Standards of Practice for Case Management* (pp. 12, 13, 27–28). Case Management Society of America.

Gillingham, D. (2020). *CCM Certification Made Easy* (3rd ed.). Blue Bayou Press.

Chapter 16

Employee Benefits Security Administration; United States Department of Labor. (2018). An Employer's Guide to Group Health Continuation Coverage Under COBRA. In *U.S. Department of Labor*. https://www.dol.gov/sites/dolgov/files/ebsa/about-ebsa/our-activities/resource-center/publications/an-employers-guide-to-group-health-continuation-coverage-under-cobra.pdf

*Health insurance rights & protection*s. (2018). HealthCare.gov; Centers for Medicare and Medicaid Services. https://www.healthcare.gov/health-care-law-protections/

Job Accommodation Network. (2018). *About JAN*. https://Askjan.org/About-Us/Index.cfm; Office of Disability Employment Policy. https://askjan.org/

Mental health and substance abuse health coverage options. (2019). HealthCare.gov; Centers for Medicare & Medicaid Services. https://www.healthcare.gov/coverage/mental-health-substance-abuse-coverage/

The Mental Health Parity and Addiction Equity Act (MHPAEA) / CMS. (2010). Cms.gov; Centers for Medicare and Medicaid Services. https://www.cms.gov/CCIIO/PROGRAMS-AND-INITIATIVES/OTHER-INSURANCE-PROTECTIONS/MHPAEA_FACTSHEET

U.S. Department of Justice Civil Rights Division Disability Rights Section. (2020, February). *A Guide to Disability Rights Laws*. www.ada.gov. https://www.ada.gov/cguide.htm#anchor62335

U.S. Department of Labor. (2009). *FMLA (Family & Medical Leave) / U.S. Department of Labor*. Dol.gov. https://www.dol.gov/general/topic/benefits-leave/fmla

Part 4: Principles of Case Management Practice

Outcomes

Readers will be able to:

- Identify ways to advocate for clients and clients' families and/or family caregiver
- Describe how to empower clients
- Identify ways to increase client activation and engagement
- List three ways to increase adherence to the care regimen
- Describe the use of evidence-based practice guidelines, standards of care, and clinical pathways

Part 4: Principles of Case Management Practice

Chapter 17

Advocacy

According to CMSA's Standards of Practice, advocacy is one of the ways case managers assist their clients to reach wellness and autonomy. The standard on advocacy states the professional CM should advocate for the client as well as the client's family or family caregiver, at the service delivery, benefits administration, and policy-making levels (CMSA, 2016).

To advocate for your client, you must first believe he has the right to self-determination in his healthcare decisions. Instead of "treating" the patient, CMs partner with them. The CM's role is not to instruct the client on what to do. Instead, CMs communicate with clients to help them determine their own goals for treatment, health, and wellness and to educate them so they can make informed decisions on how to reach those goals.

Case managers fulfill their obligation to advocate for their clients throughout the case management process. It starts with the case management assessment. During the initial assessment, as well as follow-up communications, CMs take the time to get to know the client and family, what is important to them, their goals, and barriers keeping them from meeting those goals. This allows them to see opportunities to advocate for the client when they arise.

During the planning and implementation phase of the case management process, CMs advocate for the client by creating a case management plan of care that aligns with the goals and wishes of the client. They then implement that plan of care and facilitate the client's access to necessary and appropriate services.

CMs advocate for clients by educating other stakeholders, including members of the healthcare team and the client's family and support system, about the client's needs, goals, and wishes to ensure they are honored.

At times the goals and decisions of the client will conflict with those of his family. Family support is important to clients, and in the case where the family is also the caregiver, their buy-in is necessary. There are many ways to assist in these situations and advocate for the client as well as the family. Depending on the situation, provide education, communication, and/or assist with negotiation. The goal is to find a solution that leaves everyone feeling comfortable. This is one of many instances where it's essential to utilize problem-solving and negotiation skills.

CMs need a working knowledge of a variety of topics so that they can educate the client and be strong client advocates. Examples of these topics include:

- Providers, services, programs, and resources available as well as admission, acceptance, and eligibility criteria.
- Relevant laws and regulations that may impact their client.

It is important to note that while the CM handles many tasks for clients, it's imperative to aid and empower the client to be as independent as possible. The CM may educate the client regarding a community resource available, but the application process is the responsibility of the client. There are times when the client is truly unable to do for themselves, but whenever possible, be an educator and facilitator encouraging self-care management and self-advocacy.

> Reflect on your healthcare career and create a list of times that you have advocated for your patients.
>
> Write out 2-3 detailed examples. Then save these for use in your future interview for a case management position.

Chapter 18

Self-Care Management, Self-Advocacy, and Client Adherence

Client Empowerment

The CMSA lists empowering the client as one of the roles and functions CMs perform (CMSA, 2016). A CM empowers clients, as well as family and/or caregiver(s), through support and education so they can understand and access quality, efficient healthcare.

When the CM provides education on treatment options, community resources, insurance benefits, psychosocial concerns, and the role of the CM, all stakeholders, e.g., the client, caregiver, and healthcare delivery team, can better problem solve and explore options of care to achieve the desired outcomes. The empowered client is able to manage his care and practice self-advocacy, increasing adherence to the plan of care.

Clients are empowered when they have the knowledge and resources to self-manage and self-advocate. This can be fostered by educating the client, as well as by providing information and resources to the client.

Client Self-care Management

Self-management refers to the behaviors and decisions one makes that affect their health. Self-management support is the care, education, and encouragement provided to help individuals manage their health on a daily basis, make informed decisions about care, engage in healthy behaviors, and direct their care. It involves collaboration between the client and the CM to foster ownership by the client (Pearson et al., 2007).

Shared decision-making between the provider and the patient requires the patient to be informed. Informed decision-making requires two-way communication between the patient and provider, where the patient's unique situation, beliefs, and priorities are discussed alongside the treatment options, so the patient can make the best treatment choice. It supports the ethical principle that the patient has the right to decide what care is appropriate for him, including the right to accept or decline healthcare.

Case managers empower patients to be informed and active decision-makers in their health care. They encourage patients to practice self-advocacy by explaining treatment options and providing education on the disease or injury, community resources, and insurance coverage. CMs never decide for the client, but rather guide the client in decision-making.

Client Engagement

Improved client engagement has been shown to result in better health outcomes, better quality of care, and improved patient safety. Client engagement has such an impact on health outcomes that the Affordable Care Act (ACA) has identified it as an integral component of quality in accountable care organizations (ACOs) and patient-centered medical homes. Client engagement involves the exchange of information between the client and provider, as well as the client taking an active role in care decisions.

Factors that can impact client engagement include:
- Motivation
- Attitudes
- Beliefs
- Knowledge
- Cognitive ability
- Education
- Health literacy
- Past experiences with the health system
- Degree of self-efficacy
- Trust between patient and provider

Client engagement involves building a therapeutic relationship with the client to gain trust and maximize client involvement. The engaged client will be taking action, such as exercising regularly, taking medications as prescribed, or monitoring blood sugars.

When the client is engaged, the CM is working with him, not merely talking to him. When a client is not engaged, it can seem as though the CM is swimming against the current.

To engage the client, the CM must understand what is important to him. What are his concerns, values, beliefs, and goals? It is easier to engage the client with this information in hand. The Motivational Interview is an important tool that can be used to engage the client. This will be discussed in depth in another chapter.

Client Activation

Client activation describes the knowledge, skills, ability, willingness, and confidence a person has that allows him to become actively engaged in managing his health and health care. It is very specific to the client.

The terms 'client activation' and 'client engagement' are often confused or used interchangeably. Although they are similar, they are not the same. Client engagement builds on client activation with behaviors such as maintaining a healthy diet, exercising regularly, or obtaining preventative care.

Example: An activated client has the knowledge, skills, resources, and confidence to manage his diabetes. The engaged client monitors his blood sugars, maintains his diet, and exercises daily (Gillingham, 2020).

The Patient Activation Measure (PAM) was developed by Judith Hibbard at the University of Oregon to measure a client's activation level. Studies have shown that clients with higher PAM scores are better able to engage in their health and have better health outcomes and lower healthcare costs (Hibbard et al., 2004).

Clients with lower PAM scores are more likely to feel overwhelmed with managing their health. They are also less likely to understand and have confidence in making decisions about their healthcare. By understanding a client's level of activation, healthcare clinicians can create individualized care plans to increase activation and engagement.

Ways to increase activation include:
- Meeting clients where they are
- Personalizing care
- Educating

- Empowering
- Increasing confidence
- Breaking down actions into small, manageable steps

It is easy for patients to become dependent on their CM. Our goal, however, is to empower them to take responsibility for their health issues and to not become dependent on their CM. As healthcare professionals, we are natural caregivers and love to do things for our patients. We must understand that this is not always the best course of action. Sometimes it is easier to "just do it yourself" than to teach someone else to do it, but this creates dependency.

This is not to say we never "do things for" our clients. There are times, especially at the beginning of a case, when the client is in a crisis and truly needs us to intervene on their behalf. But it is important that as soon as possible, we begin to empower them to do things for themselves. This starts with education. As the client begins to understand their situation and what they need to do and why, they can develop the confidence they need to take responsibility for their health. You can also build confidence in the client by acknowledging all the things that they are doing correctly and how far they have come. Let them know that you are confident they can or are managing their health issues.

Remember each client and situation is different. Some clients will want to take ownership and responsibility right away, others are comfortable being dependent and will want you around forever! For the latter, it is helpful to set clear boundaries from the beginning, letting them know that you are there to help them help themselves. Break actions down into small, manageable steps, and hold them accountable for accomplishing them.

Adherence to Care Regimen

Clients who are engaged and activated are more likely to adhere to their care regimen. A study over 50 years showed that on average, there is a 25% rate of nonadherence to treatment plans (DiMatteo, 2004). Nonadherence means not carrying out the treatment plan or carrying it out incorrectly. This includes the failure to keep appointments, follow lifestyle changes, maintain dietary changes, and take medication as prescribed.

It is estimated that the cost of nonadherence is $100-300 billion annually (McGuire & Iuga, 2014). In addition to the financial implications, there are clinical implications, such as decreased quality of life and premature death. CMs perform the important task of monitoring for and increasing patient adherence to care regimens.

Poor adherence to the care regimen leads to:

- Decreased quality of life
- Higher healthcare costs
- Increased emergency department visits
- Increased hospitalizations
- Avoidable nursing home admissions
- Decreased productivity
- Poor clinical outcomes
- Premature death

Conversely, improved patient adherence leads to better health outcomes, better chronic care management, improved population health, improved quality of life and productivity, and lower healthcare costs. Patient adherence is especially important for the long-term management of chronic diseases, such as kidney disease, heart disease, and diabetes.

There are numerous reasons for patient nonadherence, both intentional and unintentional. In some cases, the patient feels the care regimen is too bothersome, complex, or unnecessary. In other instances, there may be poor communication between the patient and the healthcare provider, poor health literacy leading to misunderstanding of the care regimen, or social determinants of health such as lack of transportation to carry out the treatment plan.

It is also not uncommon for patients to forget portions of what they were told by the provider. The medical industry is becoming increasingly complex, often leading to complex treatment plans. The more complex the treatment plan, the less likely a patient will adhere to it.

CMs can increase adherence to the care regimen in several ways. The first is to assess the client's knowledge and understanding of his condition and care regimen. A client's adherence can be directly correlated to his understanding.

Next, get to know the client and develop a trusting relationship with him. Client knowledge alone is not enough to increase adherence, especially when dealing with complex care regimens. Understanding the client's beliefs, attitudes, support system, social determinants of health, physical limitations, barriers, and self-efficacy will foster collaboration with the client.

CMs can begin to educate and support the client once there is a better understanding of what the client needs to know, what will motivate the client to adhere to the care regimen, and any potential barriers to adhering to the care regimen.

For effective education:

- Use simple language, avoiding medical jargon
- Limit instructions to 3-4 major points during each discussion
- Understand how the client learns best (Are they a visual, auditory, read/write, or kinesthetic learner?), and use that method whenever possible
- Supplement teaching with written materials when appropriate
- Involve the client's family or caregiver
- Evaluate client understanding
- Reinforce concepts previously taught

For clients with complex care regimens, CMs can use the Health Belief Model to optimize behavior change and adherence by ensuring that clients:

- Perceive themselves to be at risk due to lack of adoption of healthy behavior (perceived susceptibility)
- Perceive their medical conditions to be serious (perceived severity)
- Believe in the positive effects of the suggested treatment (perceived benefits)
- Have channels to address their fears and concerns (perceived barriers)
- Perceive themselves as having the requisite skills to perform the health behavior (self-efficacy)

Tailor interventions to meet the needs of the client by gaining a thorough understanding of which of these beliefs is lacking. Another important tool to increase adherence is the Motivational Interview. Both of these will be discussed further in a later chapter.

Medication Adherence

Medication nonadherence for patients with chronic diseases is extremely common. It is estimated that 50% of patients who are prescribed medications for the management of chronic conditions, such as diabetes or hypertension, do not take their medications as prescribed (Brown & Bussell, 2011). This nonadherence to prescribed treatment is thought to cause at least 100,000 preventable deaths and $100 billion in preventable medical costs per year (Kleinsinger, 2018).

The consequences of medication nonadherence are vast. Not only does the patient fail to benefit from the effects of the medication, but when the prescribing physician assumes that the patient is taking the medication as prescribed, he or she may make inappropriate medication, dosage, or treatment plan changes. This can result in further complications, unnecessary interventions, or adverse health outcomes. Creating a new illness is also a risk. For example, antibiotic-resistant bacteria have emerged as a result of patients not completing the full course of antibiotics.

Nonadherence to medications takes many forms, including primary nonadherence, such as not filling the prescription, and secondary nonadherence, such as not taking the prescription as prescribed (e.g., changing the dosage or frequency, stopping before completing the course of therapy, filling the prescription but never taking the medication, skipping or missing doses, or not refilling the prescription).

Factors that often lead to medication nonadherence include:
- Side effects
- High copays or costs
- No noticeable symptoms of the disease (for example, hypercholesterolemia and hypertension do not produce noticeable symptoms)
- Multiple doses per day

To increase medication adherence, first understand why the client is nonadherent. For example, if side effects are a problem, the solution could be to take the medication with food or to change the time of day it is taken. The client or CM should discuss with the prescribing physician the inability to take the medication. An alternative medication may be prescribed, or one that counteracts the side effects.

If the client sometimes forgets to take his medication, alarms, text messages, medication boxes, apps, and other reminders may help, or it could be associated with a part of the daily routine, such as eating breakfast, going to bed, or brushing his teeth.

Reducing the number of pills or the frequency they are taken can also increase adherence. The physician may be able to prescribe a combination medication and/or extended-release medication to decrease the number of pills taken each day.

Finally, educating the client can increase adherence. Clients who understand the purpose and importance of the prescription are more likely to be adherent.

Part 4: Principles of Case Management Practice

Chapter 19

Clinical Pathways, Standards of Care, and Practice Guidelines

Introduction

Evidence-based guidelines should be utilized in case management practice when such guidelines are available and applicable. The guidelines used should be relevant and specific to the individual client (CMSA, 2016). It's essential to be knowledgeable of the standards of care that are relevant to each client's clinical condition.

Evidence-based Practice Guidelines

Evidence-based practice is the process of applying the best available research when making decisions about healthcare. Numerous professionals analyze new research information and develop practice guidelines. The guidelines give the provider and the client recommendations for screening, diagnostic workup, and treatment that are believed to provide the best outcome.

These guidelines are not meant to replace the clinical judgment of the individual provider or establish a standard of care. They are meant to be flexible and are only considered recommendations. Healthcare professionals who promote evidence-based guidelines use research evidence, along with clinical expertise and patient preferences in providing care.

It would be impossible to give a list of all of the evidence-based practice guidelines available. Also, guidelines change as new evidence is obtained. A search online will usually provide the most up-to-date information from reputable sources. Subscribing to scholarly journals, attending conferences in your area of specialty, and obtaining continuing education on conditions you frequently encounter will also keep you up to date with the latest guidelines.

Standards of Care

Where guidelines are meant to be flexible, standards are a rigid set of criteria meant to be followed under any circumstances. These practices are medically necessary for the management of a clinical condition. Again, online research will help you find the standards of care from reputable sources as well as journals, conferences, and continuing education.

Clinical Pathway

A clinical pathway provides outcome-focused care within a certain timeline. Clinical pathways develop algorithms from evidence-based guidelines, standards of care, and protocols for common diagnoses, conditions, and procedures. These algorithms are used by a multidisciplinary care team in providing care to the client. Clinical pathways standardize treatments, promote efficiency, and improve the continuity and coordination of care provided by all disciplines involved. This results in greater quality of care and decreased costs.

Items addressed on the clinical pathway may include:
- Assessment and monitoring
- Tests and procedures
- Treatments
- Consultations
- Medications
- Activity
- Nutrition
- Education
- Targeted length of stay
- Outcome criteria
- Notification for deviations

References

Chapter 17

Case Management Society of America. (2016). *Standards of Practice for Case Management* (pp. 12, 13, 27–28). Case Management Society of America.

Chapter 18

Brown, M. T., & Bussell, J. K. (2011). Medication adherence: WHO cares? *Mayo Clinic Proceedings, 86*(4), 304–314. https://doi.org/10.4065/mcp.2010.0575

Case Management Society of America. (2016). *Standards of Practice for Case Management* (pp. 12, 13, 27–28). Case Management Society of America.

DiMatteo, M. R. (2004). Variations in patients' adherence to medical recommendations. *Medical Care, 42*(3), 200–209. https://doi.org/10.1097/01.mlr.0000114908.90348.f9

Gillingham, D. (2020). *CCM Certification Made Easy* (3rd ed.). Blue Bayou Press.

Hibbard, J. H., Stockard, J., Mahoney, E. R., & Tusler, M. (2004). Development of the patient activation measure (PAM): Conceptualizing and measuring activation in patients and consumers. *Health Services Research, 39*(4p1), 1005–1026. https://doi.org/10.1111/j.1475-6773.2004.00269.x

Kleinsinger, F. (2018). The unmet challenge of medication nonadherence. *The Permanente Journal, 22*(18-033). https://doi.org/10.7812/tpp/18-033

McGuire, M., & Iuga, A. O. (2014). Adherence and health care costs. *Risk Management and Healthcare Policy, 7*, 35–44. https://doi.org/10.2147/rmhp.s19801

Pearson, M. L., Mattke, S., Shaw, R., Ridgely, M. S., & Wiseman, S. H. (2007). *Final contract report patient self-management support programs: An evaluation.* Agency for Healthcare Research and Quality; https://www.ahrq.gov/sites/default/files/publications/files/ptmgmt.pdf (Prepared by RAND Health under Contract No. 282-00-0005).

Chapter 19

Case Management Society of America. (2016). *Standards of Practice for Case Management* (pp. 12, 13, 27–28). Case Management Society of America.

Part 4: Principles of Case Management Practice

Part 5: Utilization Management and Review

Outcomes

Readers will be able to:

- Compare utilization review and utilization management
- Explain the reasons for using utilization review/management
- Identify the main types of utilization management
- Explain the utilization management process
- Write documentation supporting approval of requested services, including all necessary information
- List factors used to determine acuity and severity levels
- Identify tools used to determine medical necessity

Part 5: Utilization Management and Review

Chapter 20

UM and UR Principles and Process

The terms utilization review (UR) and utilization management (UM) are often used interchangeably; however, there is a difference. According to URAC (formerly the Utilization Review Accreditation Commission), a nonprofit organization promoting healthcare quality by accrediting healthcare organizations, UR is the review of cases after healthcare services are carried out.

URAC defines UM as "the evaluation of the medical necessity, appropriateness, and efficiency of the use of healthcare services, procedures, and facilities under the provisions of the applicable health benefits plan" (Freedman, 2006). UM describes proactive actions such as discharge planning, concurrent review, precertification, and appeals where UR is retrospective.

UM ensures the services provided are medically necessary and provided at the appropriate and least costly level of care. Although many think this is only a concern for the payer source case manager, in reality, it is the job of all CMs. As a patient advocate, CMs understand that undergoing an unnecessary service, test, or treatment is not in the best interest of the client. Most clients will have some degree of cost-sharing, whether in the form of copay, coinsurance, deductible, or benefit maximum. Ensuring costs are contained ultimately benefits the client, as well as the payer source (Gillingham, 2020).

The Centers for Medicare and Medicaid Services (CMS) state in their Conditions of Participation (CoP) for UR that hospitals must have in effect a UR plan that provides for review of services furnished by the institution and by members of the medical staff to patients entitled to benefits under the Medicare and Medicaid programs (CMS, 2015).

There are three main types of UM: prospective, concurrent, and retrospective. (Retrospective is technically UR).

Prospective reviews, or precertifications, are done prior to the elective admission or procedure to ensure the requested service is necessary, meets the criteria for coverage, and is at the appropriate level of care.

Concurrent reviews include continued stay reviews and are conducted as the care is occurring. This includes reviews for admissions that were not precertified, as well as extending the care that was precertified. Concurrent reviews are done to ensure the client is receiving the correct care in a timely and cost-effective manner.

The retrospective review is done after care has already occurred. This can occur when precertification was required but not obtained, such as in an emergency, or as an audit.

We will now look at the UM process from the payer side with notes, when appropriate, on how the requesting CM can facilitate the process. All CMs need to understand this process, as it will be used to authorize or deny requests for clients. Understanding this process helps CMs work together to obtain timely approval or denial and avoid delays in patient care.

Chapter 21

The Utilization Management Process

Step 1: Verify eligibility

Check that the patient is covered under the health plan and that this coverage is primary.

For example:
The patient may have both Medicare and insurance through his employer. The preauthorization request would go through the primary insurance first. After the primary insurance has made its determination, a claim can be filed with the secondary insurance for any remaining balance. (You will learn how to determine primary insurance in Part 11: Reimbursement Methods and Managed Care Principles.)

Requesting case manager:
Verify all insurance the client has, and which is primary. Requesting authorization from a payer source that is not primary will result in unnecessary delays.

Step 2: Verify that the requested service is a covered benefit and determine if it requires a preauthorization

Each insurance contract (not the insurance company) determines what is and is not a covered benefit. If the requested service is a covered benefit, determine if it requires preauthorization.

For example:
Bariatric surgery may be a contract exclusion, meaning it is specifically written in the insurance contract that this is not a covered procedure. In this case, the insurance

company would not pay for the surgery or any complications resulting from the surgery. If bariatric surgery is a covered benefit, it most likely needs to meet very specific criteria and would require preauthorization.

Step 3: Gather clinical information to determine if the criteria are met for this service

This information comes from the requesting provider, such as the physician's office or hospital.

For example:
Bariatric surgery may be a covered benefit if the client meets certain criteria (BMI of 40 or greater, failure to maintain weight loss with nonsurgical methods, etc.). The requesting provider will need to provide clinical documentation that the client meets these criteria. It is the responsibility of the payer source to let the provider know what information is needed to determine if criteria are met. It is the responsibility of the provider to submit the documentation.

Requesting case manager:
Asking what documentation is required and supplying only the requested documentation will expedite the clinical review process. Not supplying all requested documentation will result in a delay because the person reviewing the request will need to stop and request additional information, sending the file back to the bottom of the list. In some instances, a different person will be reviewing the documentation when the additional information is submitted, potentially resulting in more time than necessary to review the request.

By supplying unnecessary documentation, the clinical reviewer will need to sift through numerous documents to find the needed clinical information. This increases the chance that important information will be missed, again putting the process on pause. Never send the entire chart unless this is specifically requested.

Step 4: Review clinical information to determine if the criteria for medical necessity and level of care are met, and then document as per policy

Policies and guidelines, along with resources such as MCG® or InterQual®, are often used to determine if medical necessity criteria are met. These resources are tools and assist in making a determination, but do not replace clinical judgment.

Step 5: If guidelines are met, authorize and notify the requesting provider of the approval

Each organization will have its own process for approval and obtaining an authorization number.

The following steps are only completed when a request is not approved.

Step 6: If guidelines are not met, send for physician review

The physician will approve or deny it based on medical judgment and contract guidelines. If the medical director approves the request, go back to step 5 and complete the authorization process. If the medical director denies the request, a denial letter is sent. This will include the reason for denial and the appeals process.

Requesting case manager:
All denials based on medical necessity must come from a physician. The UM/UR nurse or CM is not able to deny based on medical necessity.

Step 7: If the request is denied, the patient or treating physician may appeal

The health insurance contract and/or laws will stipulate how appeals are to be handled. Follow the employer policy for denials and appeals.

Requesting case manager:
Ask for the appeals process. If the requesting physician has information that he needs to discuss with the doctor who denied the request, he can ask for a peer-to-peer review. This allows the requesting physician to speak directly with the medical director who denied the request.

If no appeal is initiated, the process ends here.

Step 8: The medical director collects additional information and reviews the case again

The medical director may also speak with the treating physician, or send the information to an independent third-party physician with expertise in the specialty area of the request.

Requesting case manager:
Resubmitting the same information that was initially submitted rarely results in the overturn of a denial during an appeal. The reason for the denial must be supplied by the payer source.

Submit information that responds specifically to that reason. If the client has a CM at the payer source, ask to speak with her and work together to determine the best way to proceed.

Reasons for Denial

A denial can be for a clinical reason or a nonclinical reason. Reasons for a clinical denial are usually related to the submitted documentation not meeting the criteria for approval. Nonclinical reasons are not related to the patient's clinical condition, but rather related to the "rules" of the contract. An example of a nonclinical denial is a contract exclusion, where the patient's insurance contract specifically excludes this service. This often includes cosmetic procedures, dental procedures, and bariatric surgery.

Documentation

Always document according to your employer's policies. Items you will want to include in your documentation include:

- Diagnosis or symptoms
- Clinical information received supporting clinical criteria are met (in most instances this will be the most recent assessment, medications, vital signs, lab values, etc. In a retrospective review it will include the information for the time being evaluated.)
- Any references used to support determination (Example: MCG 22ed Tibia/Fibula Shaft Fracture, Closed or Open Reduction ORG: S-1124 (ISC))
- Your determination

The following is an example of documentation of approval for open reduction internal fixation (ORIF).

Diagnosis: Rt Tibial Fx. X-ray- markedly displaced right tibial fracture. Procedure approved based on MCG 22ed Tibia/Fibula Shaft Fracture, Closed or Open Reduction ORG: S-1124 (ISC)
Procedure is indicated for one or more of the following:
Open or closed reduction with internal fixation indicated by one or more of the following:

- Markedly displaced fracture

Chapter 22

Identifying Acuity or Severity Levels

Factors and Tools Used to Identify Acuity or Severity Levels

The diagnosis is only one factor used in evaluating the acuity level of the patient. Other factors that may be taken into account include:

- Comorbid conditions
- The intensity of intervention needed
- Complex medical needs
- Family/social support
- Polypharmacy
- Psychological/cognitive status
- Complex treatment plans
- Number of providers involved

Determining medical necessity for a procedure or level of service is often subjective, resulting in inconsistency with approvals and denials. For this reason, many organizations use software such as MCG® or InterQual® to assist with determining the criteria to meet medical necessity. These tools were created using research and evidence-based guidelines, making the process more objective and establishing consistency. It is important to remember these are only guidelines, and the expert opinion of the nurse, physician, or another healthcare professional is an important component in determining medical necessity.

MCG® provides evidence-based care guidelines spanning the continuum of care, including:

- Ambulatory care
- Inpatient and surgical care
- General recovery guidelines
- Recovery facility care
- Home care
- Behavioral health guidelines

InterQual® Level of Care Criteria helps healthcare organizations assess the clinical appropriateness of patient services across the continuum of care. The severity of illness, comorbidities, and complications, as well as the intensity of services being delivered, guide them to the most efficient, safest level of care.

InterQual® Level of Care Criteria are available for:

- Acute care
- Acute pediatric
- Acute rehabilitation
- Long term acute care
- Subacute care and skilled nursing facility
- Home care
- Outpatient rehabilitation and chiropractic

Many employers require experience with MCG® or InterQual® for their CMs, UR, and UM nurses. We have partnered with MCG® to give you training and experience using their software. For more information on this visit **CaseManagementInstitute.com**.

References

Chapter 20

CMS. (2015). State operations manual appendix A -survey protocol, regulations and interpretive guidelines for hospitals transmittals for appendix A. In *Centers for Medicare & Medicaid Services* (pp. 365–372). Centers for Medicare & Medicaid Services. https://www.cms.gov/Regulations-and-Guidance/Guidance/Manuals/downloads/som107ap_a_hospitals.pdf

Freedman, S. (2006, January 1). *Understand the nuances of utilization review and utilization management.* Managed Healthcare Executive. https://www.managedhealthcareexecutive.com/view/understand-nuances-utilization-review-and-utilization-mangement

Gillingham, D. (2020). *CCM Certification Made Easy* (3rd ed.). Blue Bayou Press.

Part 5: Utilization Management and Review

Part 6: Care Delivery

Outcomes

Readers will be able to:

- Compare the different care settings available to the client and the level of care provided in each setting
- Identify the case manager's role in transitions of care in various settings
- Describe the discharge planning process
- Identify the various government agency regulations and requirements associated with discharge planning and transitions of care that are relevant to case management
- Differentiate between types of advance directives
- Describe the difference between hospice and palliative care
- Identify the tools used to assess for hospice appropriateness
- Assess the needs of the acutely ill and chronically ill patient.
- Identify programs and resources available to address the vocational aspects of chronic illness and disability
- Explain the challenges of patients with multiple chronic illnesses and how the case manager can impact the client
- Describe the management of patients with multiple chronic illnesses
- Describe the role of the health coach

Part 6: Care Delivery

Chapter 23

Levels of Care and Care Settings

One of the ways the CM ensures safe, quality, cost-effective care is to verify the client is at the appropriate level of care for his specific needs. This is the lowest level of care that will safely provide for the needs of the client.

CMs are also responsible for ensuring the transfer of the client to the most appropriate care setting in a safe and timely manner. To accomplish this, CMs must have a good understanding of the different care settings available to the client, the level of care provided in each setting, and the purpose and admission criteria for each care setting.

CMs must also be aware of the insurance coverage of each individual client in regard to what benefits are available and/or remaining for the current and subsequent levels of care, as well as acceptance of that insurance coverage by the receiving facility. Network status is also an important factor, as it will drastically impact the client's out-of-pocket expenses (Gillingham, 2020).

Acute Care

Acute care is the most intensive level of care, during which a patient is treated for a brief but severe episode of illness, for conditions that are the result of disease or trauma, and/or during recovery from surgery. Acute care is generally provided in a hospital by a physician and a variety of clinical personnel. Tools such as MCG® and InterQual® will help determine if the client meets admission, length of stay, continued stay, and discharge criteria. More information on these tools was covered in Part 5: Utilization Management and Review.

Long Term Acute Care Hospitals and Long-Term Care Hospitals

According to the Centers for Medicare & Medicaid Services (CMS), long term acute care hospitals (LTACH)—also referred to as long term care hospitals (LTCH) and transitional hospitals—focus on patients who stay more than 25 days on average. Many of the patients in LTACHs are transferred in from an intensive or critical care unit. LTACHs specialize in treating patients who have one or more serious conditions who may improve with time and care but are too complex to be in a skilled nursing facility (Department of Health & Human Services, 2019). Services provided in LTACHs typically include the following: respiratory therapy, ventilator weaning, extensive wound care, complex IV therapy, pain management, and adjunctive comprehensive rehab.

Inpatient Rehabilitation

Inpatient rehabilitation hospitals provide intense, multidisciplinary therapy to patients with functional loss. To qualify for this level of care, patients must be able and willing to tolerate and participate in a minimum of three hours of therapy per day, for five to seven days per week, and be considered medically stable. Clients must be cognitive enough to follow directions provided by their therapists. Additionally, they must show improvement in their function within a couple of weeks to remain at this level of care.

Rehabilitation levels will be covered in more depth in Part 7: Rehabilitation Concepts.

Skilled Nursing Facility (SNF)

SNFs offer 24-hour skilled nursing and personal care (e.g., bathing, eating, toileting). They also provide rehabilitation services, such as physical therapy, occupational therapy, and speech therapy.

Patients must be medically stable to qualify for SNF level of care. To qualify for SNF level of care for rehabilitation, the patient must also be cognitive enough to follow therapist instructions. Patients do not need to meet the minimum of three hours of daily therapy for SNF rehabilitation as they do for inpatient rehabilitation.

For SNF level of care to be covered by insurance, the patient must need care from a skilled, licensed professional, such as a nurse or therapist, daily. Examples are complex wound care and rehabilitation when a patient cannot tolerate three hours of therapy per day. SNF level of care is not covered by insurance for custodial care.

Home Health Care

Home health care provides intermittent skilled care to patients in their homes. Services such as skilled nursing, physical therapy, occupational therapy, speech therapy, medical social worker, and home health aide visits are provided by home health agencies. For a client to qualify for home health care under Medicare, he must be deemed homebound.

Homebound means:

1) the client needs the help of another person or medical equipment such as crutches, a walker, or a wheelchair to leave their home, or their doctor believes that their health or illness could get worse if they leave their home, and

2) it is difficult for the client to leave their home and typically cannot do so.

Clients who are homebound can still leave for medical treatment, religious services, and/or to attend a licensed or accredited adult daycare center without putting the homebound status at risk. Leaving home for short periods or for special non-medical events, such as a family reunion, funeral, or graduation, should also not affect homebound status. Occasional trips to the barber or beauty parlor are also permitted (United States Health Care Financing Administration, 2020, p. 42).

Hospice Care

Hospice care provides end-of-life care to patients with a terminal illness and supports their families. To qualify for hospice care, a physician must document that the patient's life expectancy is limited, usually six months or less, if the disease follows its normal course of progression. Patients who enter hospice care no longer receive aggressive treatment for their disease, but they do receive treatment for symptom management. Hospice care can be provided in any setting, including the patient's home, hospital, SNF, or a freestanding hospice facility.

The Hospice Medicare Benefit pays a daily rate based on the level of care. The levels of care include:

- Routine home care
- Continuous home care
- Inpatient respite care
- General inpatient care

Specialty Care Centers

There are a variety of specialty care facilities that treat patients with specific needs, such as burns or brain and spinal cord injuries. The availability of these will be determined by the geographic location of the client. The admission criteria will be individualized to the institution. CMs need to be aware that these exist and to investigate the resources and financial coverage available to meet the patient's specific needs (Gillingham, 2020).

Custodial Care

Custodial care assists with personal and home care, such as activities of daily living (ADLs) and instrumental activities of daily living (IADLs). This level does not require the services of a skilled or licensed provider. Custodial care can take place in the home, SNF, or assisted living facility, among other places. Medical insurance does not cover this level of care.

Alternative Care Facilities

Assisted living

Assisted living facilities provide housing and support with ADLs and IADLs to residents. Services provided often include:

- Meals
- Medication reminders
- Transportation
- Housekeeping
- Laundry
- 24-hour staff
- Personal assistance with ADLs

Assisted living facilities do not provide medical care or skilled nursing care. The cost of assisted living is not covered by medical insurance; it is paid either by the individual, his family, or if purchased, a long-term care insurance policy. Medicaid waiver programs may also cover assisted living.

Group homes

Residents of group homes are typically children or adults with chronic disabilities requiring continual assistance to complete ADLs, IADLs, or behavioral problems that make them dangerous to themselves or others. Group homes usually house fewer than eight residents who share common areas such as the kitchen, living room, and laundry facilities and are staffed by trained personnel. The residents, depending on their ability, do chores.

Residential treatment facilities

Residential treatment facilities house and provide therapy for patients with drug and alcohol addictions, emotional or behavioral problems, and/or mental illness. They are clinically focused and offer treatments such as psychoanalytic therapy, behavioral management, group counseling, family therapy, and medication management. Residents have usually been unsuccessful with outpatient treatments, but are not appropriate for an inpatient psychiatric unit.

Levels of Care for Addiction Treatment

Levels of care for addiction are based on the program's structure, including the setting, intensity, and frequency of services.

Level I: Outpatient Treatment
Less than nine hours per week of directed treatment and recovery services.

Level II: Intensive/Partial Hospitalization Treatment
Regularly scheduled sessions for a minimum of nine hours per week in a structured program, with the opportunity for the client to interact in his own environment.

Level III: Medically Monitored Inpatient
Inpatient treatment with 24-hour observation, monitoring, and treatment by a multidisciplinary staff.

Level IV: Medically Managed Intensive Inpatient
Medical and nursing services, along with the full resources of a hospital, are available on a 24-hour basis.

Community-based programs such as Alcoholics Anonymous and Narcotics Anonymous have been found to be the most successful in treating substance abuse. Inpatient hospitalization for substance abuse is not usually the preferred method of treatment.

Part 6: Care Delivery

Chapter 24

Transition of Care

Overview

Transitions of care can occur:

- Within a facility, such as when a patient is transferred from the ICU to the step-down unit
- Between facilities, such as from a hospital to a SNF or from one acute care hospital to another
- From a facility to the community, such as from the hospital to home
- Within the community, from the primary care physician to the specialist

A transitioning patient is at increased risk for an adverse outcome due to numerous reasons, including medication errors, failure to follow up on testing or procedures, lack of communication between providers, and/or not continuing prescribed treatments or therapies. Accountability—identifying who is responsible for what—is another concern.

The CM is often involved during all points of transition and is in contact with the patient, family, and providers. This puts the CM in a unique position that enables her to serve as the coordinator of transitions of care, ensuring that needed resources are obtained, appropriate information is communicated to multiple providers, and a safe transition is secured.

The Case Manager's Role in Transition of Care

CMs provide a valuable service by overseeing the proper transition to the next level of care, as well as ensuring continuity of care. The CM's role and specific tasks performed will depend on the case management practice setting. Inpatient CMs will have more responsibility during transitions of care but managed care and other CMs play an important role in assisting the inpatient CM. When all CMs involved with the patient work together as a team, the result is better patient outcomes, less duplication of services, and seamless and more timely transitions for clients.

In general, during this phase, CMs prepare the patient for discharge or transfer by coordinating communication among the client, the current provider, the subsequent provider, and caregivers. The CMs also secure durable medical equipment and/or transportation when necessary.

Discharge Planning

CMs understand discharge planning starts on admission (or sometimes before admission, as with scheduled procedures), not when the doctor writes the discharge order. This involves assessing the patient, anticipating their discharge needs, and determining the next appropriate level of care, which can be at home or in another care setting or institution. The bedside nurse can be very helpful in this process, conveying important information to the CM.

Discharge planning continues throughout the client's stay. CMs must continue to conduct ongoing assessments to identify anything that may require adjustment to the discharge plan and update the plan of care (CMS, 2015) to ensure a timely transfer to a more appropriate level of care.

When a client is expected to discharge to home, assess whether support will be needed and the availability of that support. Also, assess for any resources they will need at home. Secure durable medical equipment (DME), home health, or other services deemed necessary. At the time of discharge, ensure the patient and family understand all discharge instructions, medications, and follow-up appointments and that there are no barriers to compliance. If barriers are found, these will need to be addressed. Once again, the bedside nurse plays an important part in this process.

After a client's discharge, contact the client and/or caregiver to confirm a smooth transition. It's important to follow up regarding post-transition services that have been or are being received, reconcile medications, and assess for issues.

Intrafacility Transfers

When a client is transferred between units in a facility, poor communication can result in missed or delayed procedures, treatments, and/or medications. Depending on the case management structure at the facility, the CM responsible for the client may also change. If this is the case, a thorough handoff report should be provided to the next CM for a seamless transition. If the client is transferred to a higher level of care due to an unexpected setback, the discharge plan will need to be reevaluated.

Interfacility Transfers

Patient transfers between facilities, such as from an acute hospital to an inpatient rehabilitation or SNF, require several considerations. Information from the client's record will need to be shared with potential receiving facilities. As HIPAA regulates client information released outside a facility, a consent for the release of information should be signed by the client (this may have been done on admission). Once this is obtained, the client's information can be shared with potential receiving facilities.

Once the client is accepted by a receiving facility, the CM will begin to coordinate the transfer. This includes communicating with members of the interdisciplinary team, the receiving facility, any outside vendors as appropriate, and the client and family. A Summary of Care Record is completed and provided to the receiving facility.

After a client transfer, the CM should contact the client and/or caregiver, as well as the receiving facility, to confirm a smooth transition. The CM will ensure post-transition services are being obtained, reconcile medications if appropriate, and assess for issues.

Transfers Within the Community

Transfers within the community, such as from a primary care provider (PCP) to a specialist, are not immune to issues. This is the reason CMS has included these transitions of care among those requiring a Summary of Care Record (see more on this in the following section). A growing number of PCPs, especially those associated with large corporations, have CMs working in their office. Among other responsibilities, CMs in these roles oversee the transition of patients referred to specialists. The managed care CM can also take on this responsibility.

In addition to ensuring that the Summary of Care Record is accurately completed and sent to the specialist or receiving physician, the office CM will communicate with the client to verify understanding of the referral or transition of care. During the transition, the client will need to know who to contact with any issues or problems that may arise.

The CM continues to follow up with the client until it is established that the transition is complete and no further involvement by the referring doctor is needed. If the patient continues to be seen by the referring doctor as well as the specialist, the CM will continue to contact the patient and may also be the liaison between the PCP and specialist.

Government Agency Regulations and Requirements

Government agencies, such as The Joint Commission (TJC) and the Centers for Medicare and Medicaid Services (CMS), have requirements that must be met regarding transitions of care, including discharge from hospitals. These are updated frequently, and the CM needs to be aware of changes that impact her role. We will look at these in-depth.

Summary of Care Record

Failure to transition properly often occurs because of a communication breakdown. For this reason, CMS recommends providers issue a Summary of Care for all transitions of care or referrals.

Providers and facilities who transition their clients to another setting of care, provider of care, or refer their patients to another provider of care, should provide a Summary of Care Record for each transition of care or referral. For this purpose, the term "transition of care" is defined as the movement of a patient from one setting of care to another. A Summary of Care Record must include the following elements:
- Client's name
- Referring or transitioning provider's name and office contact information
- Procedures
- Encounter diagnosis
- Immunizations
- Laboratory test results
- Vital signs (height, weight, blood pressure, BMI)
- Smoking status

- Functional status, including activities of daily living, cognitive and disability status
- Demographic information (preferred language, sex, race, ethnicity, date of birth)
- Care plan field (at a minimum the following components must be included: problem-focus of the care plan, goal-target outcome, and any instructions that the provider has given to the patient)
- Care team, including the primary care provider of record and any additional known care team members beyond the referring or transitioning provider and the receiving provider
- Reason for the referral
- Current problem list (at minimum, a list of current, active, and historical diagnoses, but the problem list is not limited to diagnoses)
- Current medication list
- Current medication allergy list (CMS, 2015)

This transition of care summary, also known as a discharge summary in some circumstances, provides essential clinical information for the receiving care team and helps organize final clinical and administrative activities for the transferring care team. This summary helps ensure the coordination and continuity of healthcare as patients transfer between different locations. This document improves transitions and discharges, communication among providers, and cross-setting relationships, which can improve care quality and safety.

The Joint Commission (TJC) Standards

The Joint Commission has standards that accredited hospitals must meet. In relationship to discharges and transitions of care, these include:

- Before a client is transitioned or discharged from the hospital, the patient's post-discharge needs must be evaluated and arrangements made to meet those needs. This is to include patient and family education regarding care.

- The hospital must continue to reassess the patient's needs on an ongoing basis, confirming or modifying the transition/discharge plan as needed and keeping the patient informed along the way.

- Patients must be referred to providers or agencies for post-discharge service needs. The hospital is required to communicate relevant information to the provider/agency that will assume responsibility for care post-discharge.

- Hospitals must inform the patient/family about the freedom to choose providers or services post-discharge, and when possible respect the patient's choice.

- The hospital must provide patients covered under Medicare a list of Medicare participating providers for the services they require that are available in the geographical area where the patient lives. For patients covered under commercial or managed care plans, the hospital must give the patient a list of participating providers available to them.

- Prior to discharge, the hospital must educate the patient and/or family regarding the transfer or discharge to include follow-up care. The hospital is also required to complete all paperwork needed to meet accreditation standards and legal requirements, such as notice of transition or discharge.

CMS CoP-Discharge Planning

CMS develops Conditions of Participation (CoP) and Conditions for Coverage (CfC) that healthcare organizations must meet in order to begin and continue participating in the Medicare and Medicaid programs. These health and safety standards are the foundation for improving quality and protecting the health and safety of beneficiaries.

The most recent CMS standards related to transition and discharge can be found online provided by CMS in the State Operations Manual, Interpretive Guidelines for Hospitals, Medicare CoP-Discharge Planning 482.43. At the time of publication, the following link was active. Please note that these links often change, but an internet search will provide the information. https://www.govinfo.gov/content/pkg/CFR-2007-title42-vol4/pdf/CFR-2007-title42-vol4-sec482-43.pdf

Following are the discharge CoP from CMS:

- The hospital must have in effect a discharge planning process that applies to all patients. The hospital's policies and procedures must be specified in writing.

- The hospital must identify at an early stage of hospitalization all patients who are likely to suffer adverse health consequences upon discharge if there is no adequate discharge planning.

- Discharge planning evaluation.

   (1) The hospital must provide a discharge planning evaluation to the patients identified above, and to other patients upon the patient's request, the request of a person acting on the patient's behalf, or the request of the physician.

(2) A registered nurse, social worker, or other appropriately qualified personnel must develop or supervise the development of the evaluation.

(3) The discharge planning evaluation must include an evaluation of the likelihood of a patient needing post-hospital services and of the availability of the services.

(4) The discharge planning evaluation must include an evaluation of the likelihood of a patient's capacity for self-care or of the possibility of the patient being cared for in the environment from which he or she entered the hospital.

(5) The hospital personnel must complete the evaluation on a timely basis so that appropriate arrangements for post-hospital care are made before discharge, and to avoid unnecessary delays in discharge.

(6) The hospital must include the discharge planning evaluation in the patient's medical record for use in establishing an appropriate discharge plan and must discuss the results of the evaluation with the patient or individual acting on his or her behalf.

- Discharge plan.

(1) A registered nurse, social worker, or other appropriately qualified personnel must develop, or supervise the development of, a discharge plan if the discharge planning evaluation indicates a need for a discharge plan.

(2) In the absence of a finding by the hospital that a patient needs a discharge plan, the patient's physician may request a discharge plan. In such a case, the hospital must develop a discharge plan for the patient.

(3) The hospital must arrange for the initial implementation of the patient's discharge plan.

(4) The hospital must reassess the patient's discharge plan if there are factors that may affect continuing care needs or the appropriateness of the discharge plan.

(5) As needed, the patient and family members or interested persons must be counseled to prepare them for post-hospital care.

(6) The hospital must include in the discharge plan a list of home health agencies (HHA) or SNFs that are available to the patient, that are participating in the Medicare program, and that serve the geographic area (as defined by the HHA) in which the

patient resides, or in the case of an SNF, in the geographic area requested by the patient. HHAs must request to be listed by the hospital as available.

(i) This list must only be presented to patients for whom home health care or post-hospital extended care services are indicated and appropriate as determined by the discharge planning evaluation.

(ii) For patients enrolled in managed care organizations, the hospital must indicate the availability of home health and post-hospital extended care services through individuals and entities that have a contract with managed care organizations.

(iii) The hospital must document in the patient's medical record that the list was presented to the patient or to the individual acting on the patient's behalf.

(7) The hospital, as part of the discharge planning process, must inform the patient or the patient's family of their freedom to choose among participating Medicare providers of posthospital care services and must, when possible, respect patient and family preferences when they are expressed. The hospital must not specify or otherwise limit the qualified providers that are available to the patient.

(8) The discharge plan must identify any HHA or SNF to which the patient is referred in which the hospital has a disclosable financial interest, as specified by the Secretary, and any HHA or SNF that has a disclosable financial interest in a hospital under Medicare. Financial interests that are disclosable under Medicare are determined in accordance with the provisions of Part 420, Subpart C, of this chapter.

- Transfer or referral. The hospital must transfer or refer patients, along with necessary medical information, to appropriate facilities, agencies, or outpatient services, as needed, for follow-up or ancillary care.

- Reassessment. The hospital must reassess its discharge planning process on an ongoing basis. The reassessment must include a review of discharge plans to ensure that they are responsive to discharge needs (CMS, HHS, 2007).

Chapter 25

End-of-Life Issues

CMs can help clients and families make informed decisions regarding end-of-life care that can prevent or relieve suffering and make an impact on the associated costs. It is important to understand the client's wishes regarding end-of-life care. Once these wishes are understood, provide education on the options available to the client and ensure the client's wishes are respected. This could be in the form of a palliative care consult, hospice, and/or advanced directives such as a health care power of attorney (HCPOA), living will and/or do not resuscitate (DNR)/do not attempt resuscitation (DNAR).

Patient Self-Determination Act

The Patient Self-Determination Act (PSDA) amends titles XVIII (Medicare) and XIX (Medicaid) of the Social Security Act requiring all hospitals, SNFs, HHAs, hospice programs, and health maintenance organizations that receive Medicare and Medicaid reimbursement to recognize the living will and durable power of attorney for healthcare. Under the PSDA they must:
- Ask patients if they have an advance directive
- Inform the patient of their rights under state law to make decisions concerning their medical care
- Not discriminate against persons who have executed an advance directive
- Ensure legally valid advance directives are implemented to the extent permitted by state law

- Provide education programs for staff, patients, and the community on ethical issues concerning patient self-determination and advance directives (H.R.4449 - 101st Congress (1989-1990): Patient Self Determination Act of 1990, 1990).

Advance Directives

Advance directives come in two forms, those that dictate the kind of medical treatment to be given or withheld, such as a living will or DNR, and those that appoint an agent or proxy to make healthcare decisions. Both forms only go into effect if the person is unable to make the decision for themself. Every state has its own advance directive forms and requirements. Next is a description of the different types of advance directives available. It is important to note the names may vary slightly between states and organizations.

Living will

A living will states which specific medical treatments the designated person would like to receive or have withheld. These treatments can include, but are not limited to:

- Mechanical ventilation
- Dialysis
- Tube feedings
- IV fluids
- Antibiotics
- CPR

Health care power of attorney

This type of advance directive stipulates who is to make healthcare decisions for the person if they are unable to make decisions for themselves.

Do Not Resuscitate/Do Not Attempt Resuscitation/Allow Natural Death

The do not resuscitate (DNR), do not attempt resuscitation (DNAR), or allow natural death (AND) are other types of advance directives that are a request not to have CPR and/or other types of medical interventions attempted.

Hospice Care

Hospice provides comprehensive end-of-life care and support to terminally ill clients and their families. The care provided by hospice extends beyond the patient's death by providing bereavement support for the family. To qualify for hospice care, a physician must document that the patient's life expectancy is limited, usually six months or less, if the disease follows its normal course of progression.

Hospice care is a team approach, coordinated by a CM. A hospice medical director, home health aide, social worker, chaplain, and others are all involved with the plan of care. Hospice care also covers medications related to the hospice diagnosis and DME. Room and board and treatment to cure the disease are not covered benefits for hospice.

Hospice care can be provided in an inpatient setting, such as a hospital or a freestanding hospice facility, or the home. "Home" is wherever the patient lives and does not need to be a traditional home; it can be an assisted living facility, nursing home, homeless shelter, or any other place the patient calls home.

The hospice CM's goals are unique to each client, but frequently include:
- Control pain and other symptoms for a better quality of life
- Provide information needed to make informed decisions regarding treatment and the plan of care to ensure the client has a dignified death
- Coordinate and facilitate care

A DNAR is not necessary before enrolling in hospice, but patients and families are educated on this topic, with the goal of having the DNAR in place before a patient's death.

Tools used to assess for hospice appropriateness

Karnofsky Performance Scale - Measures performance status on a scale of 0-100%, with 0 being dead and 100 being normal with no complications. A score of less than 70% (cares for self, but is unable to carry on normal activities or work) can be one of the criteria for hospice.

Eastern Cooperative Oncology Group (ECOG) - Performance status scale using a 0-4 scale with 0 being fully active and 4 completely disabled.

Palliative Performance Scale - Uses five observer-rated domains (ambulation, activity level/evidence of disease, self-care, intake, and level of consciousness) correlated to the Karnofsky Performance Scale (0-100). It is a reliable tool that aids in determining appropriateness for hospice, especially for cancer patients.

Palliative Care and Symptom Management

Many people use the terms palliative care and hospice interchangeably, but there are important distinctions. Palliative care can be employed with a patient at any stage of a severe illness. It can be used concurrently with curative treatment and is not dependent on prognosis. Alternatively, hospice care provides comprehensive care, including palliative care, for terminally ill patients with a limited life expectancy, who are no longer receiving curative treatment.

Palliative care is specialized medical care for patients suffering from serious and chronic illnesses, such as cancer, heart failure, COPD, kidney failure, and ALS, just to name a few (Center to Advance Palliative Care, 2019). The goal of palliative care is for the client and his or her family to maintain the best quality of life possible, by managing symptoms such as pain, fatigue, dyspnea, constipation, nausea, anorexia, and depression. Palliative care can be given alongside other medical treatments, such as chemotherapy and radiation, and can improve the ability to tolerate those treatments.

Palliative care is a team approach, with the core team including the doctor, nurse, and social worker. Other members may be brought into the team as needed, including a pharmacist, dietitian, massage therapist, or music therapist, among others. The palliative care team works together with the patient's other doctors and providers to anticipate, prevent, and treat suffering. The majority of palliative care today is provided by hospice, although there are palliative care specialists and practices.

The main goal of palliative care is symptom management to allow the best quality of life for the patient. To achieve this, some medication dosages and routes of administration may be different from the standard. It is also not uncommon for medications to be used off-label. For example, anticonvulsants may be used to treat pain, or morphine to ease dyspnea.

Chapter 26

Management of Acute and Chronic Illness and Disability

Acute diseases are characterized by a rapid onset with a short duration. Appendicitis, flu, pneumonia, acute respiratory distress syndrome, and acute renal failure are examples of acute illnesses. In contrast, chronic diseases require a lifetime of management, such as diabetes, lupus, heart failure, and chronic renal failure.

Acute disease may lead to chronic disease. Take, for example, a patient with acute onset of multisystem organ failure requiring a ventilator and dialysis. If the patient is unable to wean from the ventilator or if kidney function does not return, the patient has developed a chronic condition.

In managing a client with acute illness, assess whether the patient will be able to return directly to his prior level of function and living arrangement. Additionally, assess for any needs the client may have upon discharge, such as home health care or durable medical equipment. If the client is unable to return home directly from the hospital, the CM facilitates transfer to inpatient rehabilitation, LTACH, SNF, or another suitable facility.

Clients with a chronic disease must be taught to manage their condition to prevent morbidities and comorbidities. This includes medication management, lifestyle and dietary changes, and testing and follow-up with their healthcare provider. Education on self-care includes the benefits of treatment and the risks of noncompliance. They must understand their chronic diseases will not be cured, but rather managed, so they can have a better quality of life.

Healthcare professionals who specialize in helping clients manage their chronic diseases may have the title Disease Manager or Health Coach. Health coaching is secondary prevention, meaning that the client already suffers from a chronic disease. The goal of health coaching is to lessen the impact of the disease.

Health coaching uses a coordinated and proactive approach to managing care for patients with chronic illness. Health coaches, or disease managers, take on a different role than traditional medical professionals. Rather than instruct patients on what they should do, health coaches work with patients to identify and achieve their healthcare goals. The role of the health coach is to support, encourage, and empower patients to achieve their goals using evidence-based guidelines. Outcomes measured in health coaching include decreased emergency department visits and hospitalizations, adherence to guidelines, and/or clinical measures such as maintaining blood pressure or Hemoglobin A1c levels within a normal range. Successful disease management results in a higher quality of life, lower healthcare costs, and clinical improvement for the client.

Acute illness, chronic illness, and disability are all disruptions to the client's and family's lifestyle. Family members may have to take on additional responsibilities and/or rely on support systems. CMs may make referrals to support groups, counselors, financial resources, and/or disease-based agencies.

Vocational Aspects of Illness and Disability

The vocational aspects of an illness or disability can be a challenge to manage. Along with medical and psychological issues, the reduction or loss of income can place a huge burden on the client and his family. Clients usually exhaust any paid time off first. If the client is expected to be out of work for an extended period, he will want to apply for protection under the Family and Medical Leave Act (FMLA). FMLA is not a source of income, but it does protect the employee's job.

Workers' compensation clients have an advantage over clients who suffer from an illness: They are afforded benefits to get them through. Persons who are injured outside of work or suffering a prolonged illness can lose their medical and other benefits, as well as their income, if they cannot return to work or be approved for disability.

According to the U.S. Department of Health and Human Services, the employment rate for adults with disabilities is significantly lower than for those without disabilities (U.S. Bureau of Labor Statistics, 2021). The most frequently reported reasons for difficulty in obtaining employment are lack of available, appropriate jobs, followed by lack of transportation. Many individuals need some accommodation, such as accessible parking or transportation, elevators, or specially designed workstations.

The Ticket to Work Program exists for clients aged 18 to 64 who want to return to work, but currently receive Social Security benefits based on disability under the Social Security Disability Insurance (SSDI) program and/or the Supplemental Security Income (SSI) program. It is a voluntary program that provides expanded options for accessing employment services, vocational rehabilitation services, or other support services needed to enter, maintain, and advance in employment. These services include training, career counseling, vocational rehabilitation, job placement, and ongoing support services necessary to achieve a work goal. The ultimate goal of the program is to eliminate the need for Social Security disability cash benefits while allowing the client to maintain his or her Medicare or Medicaid benefits (Ticket to Work, n.d.).

Part 6: Care Delivery

Chapter 27

Management of Clients with Multiple Chronic Illnesses

Healthcare for individuals with multiple chronic conditions represents our nation's most costly (Gerteis et al., 2014) and complex healthcare, which means it is the perfect place for impactful case management intervention. These clients often receive care and information from multiple providers and care settings. This can lead to information overload and confusion about their treatment plans as they learn how to manage multiple conditions. Treatments should be coordinated by a single provider or team that understands the client's complex care needs.

Clients with multiple comorbidities are typically prescribed medications from multiple providers. This can sometimes result in overmedication or medication interactions. For this reason, CMs should review all medications upon opening the case, after each hospitalization, and after each visit to the doctor's office, at a minimum.

CMs also need to screen for medication compliance. There are numerous reasons for noncompliance, but one common reason in clients with comorbidities is the cost. These patients have significant healthcare needs, and therefore high healthcare costs. The out-of-pocket cost of their care, including the cost of prescription drugs, can be devastating. If this is the case, CMs can suggest the patient explore several options:

- Medication samples from the doctor's office
- Generic drugs when appropriate
- Co-pay assistance programs
- Disease-specific financial assistance

When multiple comorbidities are present, it can be difficult to know where to start. In some cases, one condition is extremely critical or complex, making it obvious where to start. Examples include a recent diagnosis of cancer, end-stage disease, or severely symptomatic disease. In the absence of a clinically dominant condition, concordant conditions are a good place to start. These conditions have the same overall pathophysiologic risk profile and are more likely to require similar management plans. Examples of concordant conditions are hypertension, coronary artery disease, peripheral vascular disease, and diabetes.

At times, one disease complicates the management of other comorbid conditions. In these cases, this disease must be brought under control before other conditions can be successfully dealt with. For example, a client who is severely depressed may not be able to make lifestyle changes or even keep doctor appointments. In this case, the first step is to treat the diagnosis of depression.

If none of the above circumstances apply, it is best to start where the client feels most likely to have success. Clients can be easily overwhelmed by all the information available to them. Instead of providing all the education and resources at once, ask patients what information they would like to start with first. Additional education and resources can be added with each interaction.

No matter where you start, remember patients with multiple comorbidities often require numerous lifestyle changes, as well as dietary changes or restrictions. It is often overwhelming for the patient to work on everything at once. To start, identify no more than two to three initial goals that the client feels he can accomplish. Then, commend even the smallest achievements and focus on what the client is doing right. This will build a foundation for future success.

References

Chapter 23

Department of Health & Human Services. (2019). What are Long-Term Care Hospitals? In *Medicare.gov* (p. 1). Centers for Medicare & Medicaid Services. https://www.medicare.gov/Pubs/pdf/11347-Long-Term-Care-Hospitals.pdf

Gillingham, D. (2020). *CCM Certification Made Easy* (3rd ed., p.). Blue Bayou Press.

United States Health Care Financing Administration. (2020). *Medicare & you 2001* (p. 42). U.S. Dept. Of Health And Human Services, Health Care Financing Administration. https://www.medicare.gov/sites/default/files/2020-12/10050-Medicare-and-You_0.pdf

Chapter 24

Centers for Medicare & Medicaid Services. (2015). Stage 2 Eligible Professional Meaningful Use Core Measures Measure 15 of 17 Definition of Terms. In *CMS*. https://www.cms.gov/regulations-and-guidance/legislation/ehrincentiveprograms/downloads/stage2_epcore_15_summarycare.pdf

Centers for Medicare & Medicaid Services, HHS. (2007). https://www.govinfo.gov/content/pkg/CFR-2007-title42-vol4/pdf/CFR-2007-title42-vol4-sec482-43.pdf

CMS. (2015). State operations manual appendix A -survey protocol, regulations and interpretive guidelines for hospitals transmittals for appendix A. In *Centers for Medicare & Medicaid Services* (pp. 389–412). Centers for Medicare & Medicaid Services. https://www.cms.gov/Regulations-and-Guidance/Guidance/Manuals/downloads/som107ap_a_hospitals.pdf

Chapter 25

Center to Advance Palliative Care. (2019, February 21). *What is palliative care?* Get Palliative Care. https://getpalliativecare.org/whatis/

H.R.4449 - 101st Congress (1989-1990): Patient Self Determination Act of 1990, www.congress.gov (1990). https://www.congress.gov/bill/101st-congress/house-bill/4449

Chapter 26

Ticket to Work. (n.d.). *About Ticket to Work*. Choose Work; Social Security Administration. Retrieved June 28, 2021, from https://choosework.ssa.gov/about/index.html

U.S. Bureau of Labor Statistics. (2021). Persons with a disability: labor force characteristics -2020. In *Bureau of Labor Statistics* (pp. 1–3). Labor Force Statistics. https://www.bls.gov/news.release/pdf/disabl.pdf

Chapter 27

Gerteis, J., Izrael, D., Deitz, D., LeRoy, L., Ricciardi, R., Miller, T., & Basu, J. (2014). Multiple chronic conditions chartbook 2010 medical expenditure panel survey data. In *Ambulatory care* (pp. 7–9). U.S. Department of Health and Human Services. https://www.ahrq.gov/sites/default/files/wysiwyg/professionals/prevention-chronic-care/decision/mcc/mccchartbook.pdf

Part 7: Rehabilitation

Outcomes

Readers will be able to:

- Select the rehabilitation delivery system to best meet a client's needs
- Identify the assessment of physical functioning used in rehabilitation
- Identify the different tools and resources used to assist the disabled person or injured worker to obtain or maintain employment

Following a prolonged hospitalization, orthopedic surgery, serious injury, or acute illness, clients are at risk of experiencing a significant loss of functioning. This risk is increased in clients who are critically ill, have complications, lengthy intensive care stays, disabilities or pre-existing chronic conditions, or the elderly. Early identification of rehabilitation needs and proactive rehabilitation can reduce healthcare costs.

In the event of a work-related injury, Workers' Compensation will be involved. The goal of Workers' Compensation is always to return the client to work as quickly as possible. If the client has reached Maximum Medical Improvement (MMI) and cannot perform the essential duties of the job, alternatives must be considered.

Part 7: Rehabilitation

Chapter 28

Rehabilitation Service Delivery Systems

Inpatient Rehabilitation

Inpatient rehabilitation may be provided in a medical hospital, a freestanding inpatient rehabilitation hospital, or a SNF. The setting is determined by the client's medical and functional status and the level of care the facility can provide.

The medical hospital level is for clients with an acute medical need that requires ongoing medical care. Rehabilitation such as physical therapy, occupational therapy, speech therapy, and cognitive rehabilitation is provided, but medical care is the priority. This level of care can be delivered in two hospital settings: acute care hospital or long-term acute care hospital as adjunctive therapy to an unstable condition such as ventilator weaning or complex wound care.

The inpatient rehabilitation hospital provides intense, multidisciplinary therapy to clients with a functional loss due to factors such as injury, illness, or deconditioning. The primary focus is to restore the client to self-sufficiency or maximum possible functional independence. Rehabilitation hospitals utilize an interdisciplinary team to provide intensive rehabilitation in the areas of:

- Physical therapy
- Occupational therapy
- Speech therapy
- Cognitive therapy
- Respiratory therapy

- Psychology services
- Prosthetic/orthotic services

To qualify for this level of care, clients must be able to tolerate a minimum of three hours of therapy per day, five to seven days per week, and be considered medically stable. To continue treatment the patient must participate, show ongoing progress from the initial evaluation, and continue to tolerate a minimum of three hours of therapy per day five to seven days per week.

SNFs provide rehabilitation services such as physical therapy, occupational therapy, and speech therapy, at a less intense level than inpatient rehabilitation hospitals. Patients who need rehabilitation after injury or hospitalization, but cannot tolerate three hours of therapy per day may benefit from the SNF level of rehabilitation. Patients must be medically stable to qualify for SNF care.

Community Rehabilitation

Clients who do not require the inpatient level of care can still benefit from rehabilitation services utilizing outpatient rehabilitation, clinics, or home health services.

Day program - An outpatient program for clients who no longer require hospitalization, but still need intensive coordinated rehabilitation for several hours per day.

Outpatient rehabilitation - Clients travel to a clinic or hospital to attend sessions and return home the same day. Typically a therapy session lasts from 30 minutes to an hour.

Home Health - Therapy is provided in the client's home for up to one hour per discipline per visit. Visits are usually made up to three times per week. To qualify for home health care, the patient must be homebound, meaning a taxing effort is required to leave the home. A person may leave home for medical treatment or short, infrequent non-medical reasons, such as attending religious services.

Chapter 29

Assessment of Physical Functioning

The functional assessment is an important part of rehabilitation. It guides the treatment types and duration, measures outcomes, estimates the amount of care to be provided by others, and provides documentation for payment for care. The Functional Independence Measures instrument (FIM) assesses adult inpatients, while the WeeFIM is used for children.

Functional Independence Measures Instrument (FIM)

FIM is used in the inpatient rehab setting and measures the individual's level of independence/dependence in the areas of:

- Self-care (eating, grooming, bathing, upper body dressing, lower body dressing)
- Toileting (bladder control, sphincter control)
- Transfers (bed/chair/wheelchair, toilet, tub/shower)
- Locomotion (walk, wheelchair, stairs)
- Communication (comprehension, expression)
- Social cognition (social interaction, problem-solving, memory)

Clinicians score patients from 1-7, using the following FIM Levels.

No Helper
7 - Complete Independence
6 - Modified Independence (needs the use of a device to perform safely)

Helper - Modified Dependence

5 - Supervision

4 - Minimal Assistance (Patient is able to do 75% or more)

3 - Moderate Assistance (Patient is able to do 50% or more)

Helper - Complete Dependence

2 - Maximal Assistance (Patient is able to do 25% or more)

1 - Total Assistance or not Testable (Patient is able to do less than 25%)

WeeFIM

The WeeFIM assesses children in the same areas as the FIM and uses the same rating scale. It is used for children without disabilities ages 6 months to 7 years old and in children with developmental disabilities from 6 months to 12 years old.

Chapter 30

Disability and Work-Related Injury Concepts

After a work-related injury, the goal is for the worker to achieve maximum medical improvement and to return to work as soon as possible. The return to work options are evaluated in the following order:

1. Same job, same employer
2. Modified job, same employer
3. Different job, same employer, using transferable skills
4. Same job, different employer
5. Different job, different employer, using transferable skills
6. Training for a different job with the same or different employer
7. Self-employment

The following sections will look at the various ways this is accomplished, including the use of modifications, tools, and rehabilitation programs to prepare and assist the injured worker to return to work.

Transitional Work Duty (TWS)

After a work-related injury, an employee may need some assistance before he is able to return to the job duties he had prior to the injury. If he is able to work but at a lower capacity than before the injury, the worker may be a candidate for transitional work duty (TWD). For example, this would be appropriate for a police officer who broke his leg. He is able to work, but not in his normal job function. He could be placed in a desk job until he is able to return to his normal job duties.

TWD allows an injured employee to return to productive work with their employer while under the care of rehabilitation professionals. The employer creates a value-added temporary position based on the knowledge and skills of the employee. The work must conform to the restrictions put in place by the employee's treating physician. Only employees with temporary injuries who will eventually be able to return to their normal full-time duties are eligible for TWD.

Job modification/Job accommodation

A person with a disability or work-related injury may require modification(s) or accommodation(s) to enable them to perform their job. The terms job modification and job accommodation are often used interchangeably. To differentiate, however, a job modification is an across-the-board change to the job description, targeting skills. Examples include:

- Restructuring the job
- Eliminating marginal job functions
- Sharing job duties
- Modifying company policy

Job accommodations are more individualized and focus on access. Examples include voice recognition software or an adjustable height desk to accommodate a wheelchair. Because most of the literature, as well as most CMs, use both terms interchangeably, the term accommodation will be used for the remainder of this section.

The accommodation process

- Request accommodation: The person with the disability is responsible for requesting the accommodation.

- Identify functional limitations: Determine where the functional limitations intersect with the job duties; that is, which tasks the person cannot perform without accommodation.

- Identify accommodations: Discuss options with the employee. Often the accommodation is obvious or something the employee has used before successfully, but creative collaboration, extensive investigation, or outside assistance may be needed.

- Determine reasonable solutions: The ADA requires employers to provide reasonable accommodations for qualified applicants or employees with disabilities unless doing so would cause undue hardship for the employer. Undue hardship can refer to accommodations that cause financial difficulty, are disruptive to the workplace, or fundamentally change the operation of the business (Employers' responsibilities I U.S. Department of Labor, 2019).

- Make accommodation: The employee's preferences should be taken into account, but ultimately the employer will determine which accommodation is put into effect based on cost, business feasibility, and effectiveness.

- Monitor effectiveness: If the desired outcome is not achieved, the employee and employer should start the process again.

The Job Accommodation Network (JAN) is a consulting service provided by the U.S. Department of Labor's Office of Disability Employment Policy (ODEP) that provides free information on job accommodations (Job Accommodations I U.S. Department of Labor, 2019). JAN's website states, "Working toward practical solutions that benefit both employer and employee, JAN helps people with disabilities enhance their employability, and shows employers how to capitalize on the value and talent that people with disabilities add to the workplace" (Job Accommodation Network, n.d.).

Data collected on the cost of accommodations show that more than half of all accommodations cost nothing. For modifications that do have a cost, the majority are under $500, and tax incentives and funding are available through several organizations to help offset the expense (Job Accommodation Network, n.d.).

Accommodations are not limited to adjustment or modifications of physical equipment. The ADA lists these six categories of accommodations:

1. Job restructuring - Adjustments to work procedures
2. Assistive devices - Equipment that helps the employee complete the task
3. Training - Helps an employee learn or relearn job duties
4. Personal assistant - A person who helps an employee with job duties
5. Building modification - Alterations to the physical environment that allow equal access to the facility
6. Job reassignment - Temporary or permanent transfer of task assignment, or sharing jobs with other employees

Job Analysis

Knowing the job duties of the worker's position is important in determining if and when the individual will be able to return to work and what, if any, accommodations are needed. A job analysis may be done to identify these duties.

A functional job analysis is a process of collecting data to define a person's job requirements and essential and nonessential job duties. This data can be collected from interviews with workers and supervisors, on-site observations, and analysis of company job descriptions. It provides detailed information related to major tasks, as well as the physical, cognitive, and behavioral capacities required to perform the job. Items examined in the job analysis may include:

- Essential duties of the job
- Tools and equipment used
- Amount of time spent standing, walking, sitting, operating a vehicle, climbing, reaching, bending, kneeling, and lifting
- Specific tasks
- Details regarding scheduling, location, equipment needed, and required competencies

In rehabilitation, the goal of the job analysis is to identify essential job functions and requirements to satisfactorily perform the work. Job requirements must be the focus, not the individual worker's skills. Essential job functions are the basic duties fundamental to the job, and the employee must be able to perform them with or without reasonable accommodations. The most obvious functions are those the position exists to perform. For example, an obvious job function for a cashier is to exchange money with customers. Other criteria for determining essential job functions include a reference in the written job description, the amount of time spent performing the function, and the consequences if this employee is not required to perform a particular function.

The job analysis may be performed by one discipline or an interdisciplinary rehabilitation team. Disciplines that often perform rehabilitation job analysis include:

- Physical therapists
- Occupational therapists
- Vocational rehabilitation specialists
- Ergonomists

Functional Capacity Evaluation (FCE)

The Functional Capacity Evaluation (FCE) is an important part of rehabilitation. It guides the treatment types and duration, measures outcomes, estimates the amount of care to be provided by others, and provides documentation for payment for care.

The FCE is used to directly measure the patient's physical ability to perform work-related activities. The worker is examined as he or she completes activities, directly measuring the physical level of work the individual can perform. It is a tool that is dependent on the motivation, cognitive awareness, and sincerity of effort of the participant and only reflects what he or she is able or willing to do at the time of the evaluation. Factors that may influence this include sincerity of effort, motivation, and mental alertness.

The FCE is a comprehensive exam, covering all physical demands required of the employee. It can be part of the initial assessment, used to determine a work conditioning plan, or to reassess progress and the ability to return to work. Along with assessing the capacity for returning to the current job, it can also be used to assess for a job modification or a new job. The FCE is done in a structured setting, not the place of work, and is performed by an independent physical therapist, occupational therapist, or physician, not the treating clinician.

During the FCE the client is evaluated as he performs activities required for his job. This may include, but is not limited to:

- Squatting
- Sitting
- Pushing
- Pulling
- Turning
- Standing
- Kneeling
- Balancing
- Navigating stairs
- Handgrip

The amount of time the client requires to perform each of these tasks is also important.

Work Hardening, Work Conditioning, and Work Adjustment

An employee who has recovered from his or her injury may need work conditioning or work hardening to be able to return to pre-injury duties. These therapies are ideal for patients who have already progressed through traditional physical therapy but still lack full function in relation to the specific job duties required.

Work hardening is an individualized, intense, highly structured program designed to return the worker to full employment in a safe and timely manner. It focuses on work endurance by progressively increasing tolerance with conditioning exercises including strength, flexibility, and spine and joint stabilization exercises. It can also include job task training such as pushing, pulling, bending, twisting, or lifting. The hardening ensures that muscles are conditioned specifically for the job-related tasks to be undertaken by the worker. The program is individualized to the client based on his or her injury or impairment and job description. Job analysis or on-site observation of the worker's job may be performed to identify goals related to job functions.

Work conditioning aims to restore function so the client can return to work. It is done under the direction of a physical therapist in a therapy setting two to four times per week. Work conditioning differs from work hardening in that the focus is not on specific tasks the client must perform (for example, lifting a 20-pound box and placing it on a shelf), but rather on building the strength required to lift anything.

The focus of work adjustment is on attitude, behavioral, and social skills for clients with behavioral health issues. Work adjustment can be done individually or in a group setting. Real or simulated work activity is performed under close supervision at a rehabilitation facility or in the work setting. The goal is to improve problems that prevent the client from obtaining employment, such as attendance, punctuality, hygiene, or interpersonal relationship skills. Work adjustment might be used after a traumatic brain injury, for example, wherein the worker has developed behavioral issues.

Transferable Skills Analysis

If the client has reached Maximum Medical Improvement (MMI) and cannot perform the essential duties of the job, with or without accommodation, a Transferable Skills Analysis can be completed to document current and projected employment based on the skills, abilities, and aptitude of the client. A Vocational Evaluation can be completed to determine the client's work capacity and potential for vocational rehabilitation.

If the medical or Workers' Compensation CM determines the client may need vocational case management (vocational rehabilitation) to assist with job development or placement after an injury, he or she should make or obtain the referral. The vocational CM will then create a vocational rehabilitation plan to assist the client in obtaining employment.

References

Chapter 30

Employers' responsibilities | U.S. Department of Labor. (2019). Dol.gov; U.S. Department of Labor. https://www.dol.gov/general/topic/disability/employersresponsibilities

Job Accommodations | U.S. Department of Labor. (2019). Dol.gov; U.S. Department of Labor. https://www.dol.gov/general/topic/disability/jobaccommodations

Job Accommodations Network. (n.d.). *Frequently Asked Questions*. Askjan.org; Office of Disability Employment Policy. Retrieved June 29, 2021, from https://askjan.org/Frequently-Asked-Questions.cfm

Part 8: Psychosocial Concepts and Support Systems

Outcomes

Readers will be able to:

- Identify the impact the social determinants of health have on individuals

- Assess clients for social determinants of health

- Describe interventions case managers may implement to address social determinants of health

- Demonstrate cultural competence when managing clients

- Create case management plans of care that respect their client's spiritual and cultural beliefs

- Explain the importance of including a cultural and spiritual assessment as part of the initial case management assessment

- Identify ways the information obtained during the spiritual and cultural assessment impacts the case manager's plan of care

- Compare the behavioral change theories case managers use and how they apply to case management

- Determine the client's health belief as related to the Health Belief Model and use this information to determine where to focus efforts to induce change

- Identify the stage of change a client is in and the best way to support the client to move into the next stage of change

- Summarize the key concepts of the motivational interview

- Describe the psychosocial impact a chronic illness or disability has on the client

- Identify factors that influence a client's self-efficacy, as well as actions to foster and encourage self-efficacy in the client

- Identify the role family dynamics play in case managing a client

- Distinguish between an adaptive family and a maladaptive family

- Identify various types of abuse and neglect that may be encountered when case managing a client

- Describe interventions that can reduce the likelihood of abuse and neglect

- Differentiate between substance use and abuse

- Assess a client for substance use disorder

- Define dual diagnosis

- Describe interventions to implement that can assist the client in crisis

Chapter 31

Social Determinants of Health

The Centers for Disease Control and Prevention (CDC) lists five factors that contribute to a person's current state of health:

- Biology and genetics (sex, age)
- Individual behavior (alcohol use, injection drug use, unprotected sex, smoking)
- Social environment (discrimination, income, gender)
- Physical environment (where a person lives, crowding conditions)
- Health services (access to quality healthcare, health insurance status) (2019)

Biology and genetics are fixed, but the remaining factors can be modified and together are known as the social determinants of health (SDH). The World Health Organization (WHO) defines SDH as the conditions in which people are born, grow, live, work, and age (*Social determinants of health*, 2020). The SDH are the factors that affect health outside of the hospital and doctor's office and include, but are not limited to housing, social services, geographical location, and education.

Examples of social determinants include:

- Availability of resources to meet daily needs (e.g., safe housing and local food markets)
- Access to educational, economic, and job opportunities
- Access to health care services
- Availability of community-based resources in support of community living and opportunities for recreational and leisure-time activities

- Transportation options
- Social support
- Socioeconomic conditions (e.g., concentrated poverty and the stressful conditions that accompany it)
- Language/literacy
- Access to mass media and emerging technologies (e.g., cell phones, the Internet, and social media)
- Exposure to toxic substances and other hazards
- Infrastructures, such as buildings, sidewalks, bike lanes, and roads

Let's take a closer look at how the SDH may impact the clients we serve. We know that poverty is a factor that can limit access to healthy foods, safe living conditions, and access to care, but it is important to remember, even where poverty is not a factor, SDH impact the health of our clients. For example, a shortage of providers and specialists in the geographical area may result in long waits to access healthcare. Rural areas may not have the transportation options necessary for clients to access healthcare. Rural areas may also lack a public water source leaving residents using underground water sources that are potentially contaminated.

Healthy People (HP) is a national effort led by the U.S. Department of Health and Human Services (HHS) to identify and set science-based goals and objectives to improve the health and well-being of people living in the United States in a 10 year period. Healthy People 2030 (HP2030) was launched in August of 2020 and is the fifth iteration of the initiative. Much of the research, goals, and objectives are based on the social determinants of health. We will be referencing HP often as we take a deep dive into a few of the social determinants that impact the health of our clients.

Access to Healthcare

HP2030's extensive research surrounding access to health services and primary care (Office of Disease Prevention and Promotion, n.d.-b) found that many people face barriers that prevent or limit access to needed healthcare services, such as lack of health insurance, poor access to transportation, and limited health care resources.

Specific findings related to access to healthcare include:

- Uninsured adults may delay seeking care when they are ill or injured, are more likely to be hospitalized for chronic conditions such as diabetes or hypertension, and are less likely to receive preventive services for chronic conditions such as diabetes, cancer, and cardiovascular disease.

- Uninsured children are less likely to get vaccinations or routine primary care services, and less likely to receive appropriate treatment for conditions like asthma.

- Even for those with insurance, out-of-pocket medical costs can still leave health care out of financial reach for many individuals, causing them to delay or forgo needed care (such as doctor visits, dental care, and medications).

- Transportation barriers can lead to delaying or skipping medications, rescheduling or missing appointments, or postponing care, and have been associated with the late-stage presentation of certain medical conditions (e.g., breast cancer).

- Limited availability of healthcare resources, such as physician shortages or a limited number of physicians who accept Medicaid due to their reduced reimbursement rates.

- Individuals living in rural areas may not have easy access to hospitals, pharmacies, dialysis clinics, physicians, and other healthcare resources.

Speaking a language other than English at home can also impact access to healthcare. For example, a study found that Hispanic individuals who did not speak English at home were less likely to receive recommended preventive healthcare services for which they were eligible (Cheng et al., 2007). Another study examined women of various racial and ethnic groups whose primary language was not English (they spoke Spanish, Cantonese, or Japanese) and found they were less likely to be screened for breast or cervical cancer (Jacobs et al., 2005).

Another barrier to accessing healthcare is hours of availability. Most physicians' offices, testing centers, and clinics have limited office hours, which may coincide with the work hours of the client. For a worker without sick leave benefits, missing work for a medical visit can result in lost wages, or worse, losing their job.

Access to Foods that Support Healthy Eating Patterns

Studies show a relationship between the inability to access foods that support healthy eating patterns and negative health outcomes. One study of 40,000 California residents looked into how access to healthy food choices impacts rates of obesity and diabetes. Residents of neighborhoods with fewer fresh produce sources, plentiful fast-food restaurants, and many convenience stores were at a higher risk of developing obesity and diabetes (Babey et al., 2008, as cited in Healthy People 2020).

Low-income groups tend to rely on foods that are cheap and convenient to access but are often low in nutrient density. Fresh fruits, vegetables, and other healthier items are often more expensive at convenience stores and small food markets than in larger chain supermarkets and grocery stores. A summary of research on this issue indicated that "in neighborhoods without supermarkets, residents likely face higher prices for many healthy foods because small stores typically charge more for items such as fresh produce" (Rose, 2010, as cited in Healthy People 2020). Research also shows that price reductions of healthier food choices can contribute to increased purchasing of those choices (French, 2003, as cited in Healthy People 2020).

The distance to the nearest supermarket or supercenter for the average U.S. household is 2.14 miles (Mentzer Morrison & Mancino, 2015). Individuals without a vehicle, access to convenient public transportation, or who do not have food venues with healthy choices within walking distance, have limited access to foods that support healthy eating patterns. This can have a serious negative impact on those living in low-income and rural communities, especially older adults living in rural communities (Sharkey et al., 2010).

Environmental Conditions

The World Health Organization attributed 11% of U.S. mortality in 2012 (over 280,000 deaths) to environmental causes (*Deaths attributable to the environment - data by country*, 2016). Contaminated water, polluted air, and extreme heat are three of the many environmental conditions that can negatively impact health.

Poor water quality places the public's health at risk. It is estimated that more than 13 million U.S. households get their drinking water from private wells. The Environmental Protection Agency (EPA) does not regulate private wells and private well owners are responsible for the safety of their water (*Private wells*, 2015). Public water sources may also contain contaminants above the recommended levels. In 2009, the EPA completed its "Six-Year Review of National Public Drinking Water Resources" and concluded that public water systems in 44 states tested at least once for arsenic at levels higher than the maximum contaminant level allowed (*Picture of American Drinking Water Fact Sheet*, n.d.).

Air quality is another factor that can influence health and includes indoor and outdoor air quality. This can be the presence of radon or mold, as well as ozone and fine particulate matter. Research has shown that children, pregnant women, older adults, and individuals with pre-existing conditions are at an increased risk of adverse effects from air pollutants (*Research on health effects from air pollution*, 2021).

HP2030's analysis of 10 studies in their report on environmental conditions (*Office of Disease Prevention and Promotion, n.d.-d*) found that:

> Air temperature is another environmental condition that affects health. According to recent reports from the National Oceanic and Atmospheric Administration (NOAA), many of the hottest years on record have occurred in the past decade. Older adults and children are at increased risk for heat-related disease and death. In addition, racial and ethnic minorities have higher rates of heat-related disease and death. This association may be due to factors such as living in urban areas, lacking air conditioners, and working in agriculture.

Housing Instability

HP2030's report on housing instability (*Office of Disease Prevention and Promotion*, n.d.-e) reviewed 34 studies and found that housing instability:

> encompasses a number of challenges, such as having trouble paying rent, overcrowding, moving frequently, staying with relatives, or spending the bulk of household income on housing. These experiences may negatively affect physical health and make it harder to access health care...
>
> Households are considered to be cost-burdened if they spend more than 30% of their income on housing and severely cost-burdened if they spend more than 50% of their income on housing. Cost-burdened households have little left over each month to spend on other necessities such as food, clothing, utilities, and health care...
>
> People with the lowest incomes may be forced to rent substandard housing that exposes them to health and safety risks such as vermin, mold, water leaks, and inadequate heating or cooling systems. They may also be forced to move in with others, potentially resulting in overcrowding...Overcrowding may affect mental health, stress levels, relationships, and sleep, and it may increase the risk of infectious disease.
>
> Moving three or more times in one year, often called "multiple moves," has been associated with negative health outcomes in children. Children who move frequently are more likely to have chronic conditions and poor physical health.

Impact for Case Managers

Individuals affected by social determinants of health (SDH) are often those that need the CM the most, as they can benefit considerably from case management services. They are the clients you will see in the emergency department repeatedly. They are the clients who will be labeled as "noncompliant" or "nonadherent" because they cannot follow the treatment plan. They are the clients who result in less than optimal outcomes for the CM and healthcare organization if SDH are not addressed. By understanding how SDH impact clients and the resources available to address them, it's possible to find creative resource solutions.

This is one of the many reasons the screening and assessment are such an important part of the case management process. A thorough assessment must include all of the domains including social, medical, functional, cognitive, and behavioral. This comprehensive assessment will allow CMs to identify any SDH that may impede the ability of the client to reach his goals. Once identified, develop a case management plan of care that addresses these barriers.

Look at each area discussed in this section and describe interventions case managers may enlist to assist clients with each barrier.

- Access to healthcare
- Access to foods
- Environmental conditions
- Housing instability

Chapter 32

Cultural, Spiritual, and Religious Factors

Cultural competency is an important part of case management, so much so that CMSA has included a standard on it in their Standards of Practice. Culture can include language, beliefs, values, traditions, foods, and customs, among other things. The CM is to be aware of, respectful of, and responsive to, the cultural diversity of clients. CMs are to take part in ongoing cultural competency training to enhance their work with multicultural populations.

A cultural assessment, including an assessment of the client's linguistic needs, should be included in the CM's initial client assessment. While it is necessary to understand general cultural norms as they relate to healthcare, it is more important to understand that each client is an individual with his own individual, family, and cultural beliefs. Sometimes these cultural beliefs conflict with the treatment plan. When this happens the CM should attempt to adjust the treatment plan to work within the client's cultural beliefs. If this is not possible, educate the client on the possible effects of not complying with the treatment plan. This should be done respectfully without coercing the client. Ultimately, it is the client who chooses to follow the treatment plan.

At times, the client's cultural beliefs may be very different from the case manager's, which can influence the client-CM relationship. Respect the client's beliefs, even though you may not agree with them. It can be helpful to acknowledge cultural differences with the client and reassure the client that your job as the CM is to provide education and support his decisions.

CMs need to assess the client's language preference and identify resources to enhance proper communication. This may include the use of interpreters and material in different languages and formats. When using an interpreter, it is best to use a professional interpreter and not a family member whenever possible (Gillingham, 2020, p. 169).

Spirituality As It Relates to Health Behavior

Spirituality is a broad concept with many perspectives. In general, it includes a sense of connection to something bigger than us, and it typically involves a search for meaning in life. For some people, spirituality is synonymous with religion, but a person can be spiritual without having a religious identity.

It is important to have an understanding of the client's spiritual and religious views, as the views often impact the choices they make regarding healthcare. For example, if a client believes he has no control over his destiny, he may feel lifestyle changes or medical intervention will not change the inevitable, and therefore decline treatment or lifestyle changes. On the other hand, if the client believes life is precious and all means should be exhausted in prolonging it, he may be unwilling to accept the withdrawal of life-sustaining treatment, even when death is inevitable. Some religious beliefs can affect health care choices. For example, Jehovah's Witnesses do not accept blood transfusions and some Pentecostal Christians will refuse medical treatment due to their strong belief in miraculous healing.

Assessing a client's spiritual needs is an important part of the initial assessment with the client. With this information, CMs are able to refer the patient to resources for spiritual counseling if indicated. During times of illness, patients often rely on their spiritual beliefs to cope. Spiritual practices tend to improve coping skills, provide optimism and hope, promote healthy behavior, decrease feelings of depression and anxiety, and encourage a sense of relaxation. By relieving stressful feelings and promoting healing ones, spirituality can positively influence the immune, cardiovascular, hormonal, and nervous systems. Studies have shown that terminally ill clients with higher spiritual well-being were less likely to have depression and thoughts of suicide.

CMs should not judge a client's spirituality-based healthcare decisions. Instead, when possible, work to find alternatives that are within the client's beliefs.

Chapter 33

Behavioral Change Theories and Stages

CMSA Standards of Practice Section IV Part B states that case managers "Promote the integration of behavioral change science and principles throughout the case management process" (Case Management Society of America, 2016).

Theories of behavior change usually involve:

- Reduction or elimination of destructive behavior
- Promotion of healthier lifestyle
- Adherence to medical regimens

In this section, we will discuss three behavioral change theories CMs use and how they apply to case management.

The Health Belief Model (HBM)

The Health Belief Model (HBM) is a psychological model that attempts to explain and predict health behaviors. This is done by focusing on the attitudes and beliefs of individuals. The HBM was first developed in the 1950s by social psychologists Hochbaum, Rosenstock, and Kegels, working in the U.S. Public Health Services. The HBM predicts that behavior is a result of a set of core beliefs, which have been redefined over the years. The core beliefs are the individual's perception of:

1. Susceptibility to illness - One's opinion of chances of getting a condition (e.g. "my chances of getting lung cancer are high")

2. The severity of the illness - One's opinion of how serious a condition and its consequences are ("lung cancer is a serious illness that can lead to death")

3. Barriers to advised action - One's opinion of the tangible and psychological cost of the advised action ("not smoking will make me irritable")

4. The benefits involved in carrying out the behavior - One's belief in the effectiveness of the advised action to reduce risk or seriousness of impact (e.g. "not smoking will lower my risk of developing lung cancer and improve my ability to play basketball without becoming short of breath as quickly")

5. Cues to action which may be internal (e.g. "the symptoms of breathlessness"), or external (e.g. information in the form of health education leaflets)

6. Self-efficacy - Confidence in one's ability to take action ("if I put my mind to it I could stop smoking")

Application for Case Managers

By assessing the client's health belief as related to the HBM, the CM will be able to determine where to focus her efforts. For example, if the client's perceived susceptibility is too low, the CM will work to increase the perceived susceptibility by focusing conversations and teaching on this area. However, if the client's perceived barriers are too high, the CM will work to identify and reduce barriers through reassurance, incentives, and/or assistance.

Health Belief	Desired Perception	Intervention to improve
Perceived Susceptibility	High	Increase clients' perceived susceptibility through education and/or motivational interviewing
Perceived Severity	High	Increase clients' perceived severity by specifying consequences of the risk and the condition.
Perceived Barriers	Low	Identify and reduce barriers through reassurance, incentives, and/or assistance.
Perceived Benefits	High	Define action to take; how, where, when; clarify the positive effects to be expected.
Cues to Action	High	Provide how-to information, promote awareness, reminders.
Self-Efficacy	High	Provide training and guidance in acting.

Stages of Change

The Stages of Change Model introduced the idea that people move through a succession of five or six relatively distinguishable stages in making behavior changes. Key features of the Stages of Change Model are:

- Only deals with intentional behavior change
- Views change as a process rather than an event
- Characterized by a series of change stages
- Those attempting to change a behavior typically cycle through these stages of change

The six stages of change are:

1. Precontemplation
2. Contemplation
3. Preparation
4. Action
5. Maintenance
6. Relapse (if this occurs)

In the precontemplation stage, the individual does not intend to take action in the foreseeable future. "I don't want to quit smoking." He may not think about the change or he may be resistant to it. Pressuring the client at this stage is usually not effective. When working with a client in this stage, express concern and ask permission to discuss the subject.

In the contemplation stage, the individual considers a change in the next six months but has not committed to it. "I know I need to quit smoking, I just don't know how." He may be open to information on the benefits of change and how to successfully do so. Elicit the client's perspective and provide information to help the client to make the decision to change.

Preparation is when the individual actively plans to make a change within the next month. They may even have taken small steps toward change. "I got my nicotine patches today and have set my quit date." Help the client prepare for the change and talk through challenges that may occur. Work together to develop a plan to decrease the impact of those challenges. For example, if the client expresses concern that he always smokes when he has a beer at the bar after work, discuss alternatives to prevent this trigger. The most obvious would be to avoid going to the bar after work. If this is not a lasting option, the client and CM would work together to develop other plans.

Action is the stage when the individual has successfully made a change and has sustained it for less than six months. He will be seeking reinforcement and encouragement. "I have not had a cigarette in nine days." Continue to support the client by congratulating them and discussing the difference between a slip and relapse. Discuss with the client any potential problems in maintaining the change, and develop action steps to prevent relapse from occurring.

When the change has been sustained for more than six months, maintenance has been achieved. Continue to provide support as needed to reduce the risk of relapse.

Relapse can occur at any level and is defined as a consistent return to a problem behavior after a period of resolution. Frame relapse as a learning opportunity in preparation for the next action stage.

Motivational Interviewing

Motivational interviewing is a collaborative, goal-oriented style of communication that pays particular attention to the language of change. It is designed to strengthen personal motivation for and commitment to a specific goal by eliciting and exploring the person's own reasons for change within an atmosphere of acceptance and compassion. Motivational interviewing was developed specifically for the purpose of helping people resolve ambivalence and strengthen motivation for change.

The four key processes in motivational interviewing are:

1. Engaging - establishing a helpful connection and working relationship
2. Focusing - developing and maintaining specific direction in the conversation about change
3. Evoking - eliciting the client's own motivations for change
4. Planning - developing a commitment to change and formulating a concrete plan of action.

Motivational interviewing avoids using the "righting reflex," the urge to want to help the client by correcting them or giving them the information they need to make the right choice. Often this is automatic, almost reflexive, for us. We are here to help them, right? And if we could just give them all of the information they would, of course, choose to change, right?

The client who is ambivalent to change sees the reasons for and against change and often has both internal conversations. By giving the client the reasons to change, he will instinctively resist and bring up all the reasons not to change. Most people trust their own opinion more than that of others. Therefore, if you are arguing for change and causing the client to verbalize the reasons against change, you are decreasing the likelihood that he will change. For this reason, it is important not to correct the client or tell them the reasons why they should change, as this will most likely put the client on the defensive. Instead, direct the conversation in a way that will allow the client to come up with and verbalize their own arguments for change.

It is appropriate to offer advice or information when the client asks for it, or if you ask for permission to do so. Remember not to use this opportunity to direct the client, but rather to give information based on the perspectives and needs of the client, helping him to reach his own conclusions.

The key communication skills used through motivational interviewing can be remembered by the acronym **OARS**:

- **O**pen questions - Questions that deliberately seek long answers. We will discuss these in-depth in the unit on communication. In motivational interviewing, we do not ask open questions to gather information, but rather to help understand the client's internal frame of reference and evoke motivation.

- **A**ffirming - Recognizing and commenting on the client's strengths, abilities, and efforts.

- **R**eflecting - Reflective statements make a guess about the client's meaning. This allows the client to hear again the thoughts and feelings he is expressing in different words. Good reflective listening keeps the client talking, exploring, and considering.

- **S**ummarizing - Summarizing is broader than reflecting in that it can be a summary of what a person has been saying, drawing together the client's motivations and intentions.

While these communication skills are necessary to practice motivational interviewing proficiently, they are not in themselves motivational interviewing. The way that these skills are strategically used to help elicit change is motivational interviewing.

Motivational interviewing can be manipulative if the underlying spirit is not correct. There are four key elements to the spirit in which motivational interviewing must be done to keep this from occurring:

1. Partnership - Motivational interviewing is not done "to" a person, but rather "with" a person.

2. Acceptance - This is not approval of the client's actions, but rather accepting their value as an autonomous person.

3. Compassion - Actively promoting the welfare of the other and ignoring your own self-interest.

4. Evocation - Motivational interviewing works on the belief that the client already has within him much of what is needed, and your task is to evoke it.

Chapter 34

Psychosocial Aspects of Chronic Illness and Disability

There is no consensus on the definition of chronic illness, but for our purposes, we are referring to clients with a health condition that at best can be controlled, but not cured. This includes, but is not limited to, diabetes, heart disease, Alzheimer's, and COPD. A disability is considered chronic when the impaired function will never be completely eliminated. It is important to remember to assess not only the physical effects of chronic illness or disability but also the psychosocial effects on both the client and his family and caregivers.

A chronic illness or disability can change the client's self-perception of his role in society, work, and family, as well as how he is perceived by others. CMs must understand the client's self-perception of his role, and how he perceives that role is affected by the illness or disability. This will help CMs understand the psycho/social impact of the illness or disability.

Many factors influence how a client perceives and responds to a chronic illness or disability, including but not limited to, the impact it has on his daily life, his family, social support network, and his coping skills. The client's level of self-efficacy also has a major impact on how well he will adjust.

Self-efficacy is one's belief in his or her own ability to succeed, and it plays a major role in the client's outcome. The more self-efficacy a client possesses, the more likely he or she will persevere when obstacles arise. For a behavioral change to take hold, the client must know what to do, believe it is beneficial, and believe it is attainable.

Factors that influence self-efficacy include the client's physiological and psychological state, mastery of experiences, vicarious experiences, and social persuasion. With each experience the client masters, he finds evidence he has the ability to succeed. Witnessing others in similar situations overcome their obstacles is further proof that perseverance can lead to success. Continuous positive persuasion strengthens personal beliefs regarding success.

Self-efficacy can be fostered and encouraged in the client in many ways. One way is by providing affirmation, motivation, and encouragement. Another is to facilitate goal setting that will promote mastery by helping the client create small, attainable goals. Many chronically ill and disabled individuals have made major contributions to society. Tell these individuals' stories to remind the client what is possible. Assist the client to reach optimal physical and psychological function by making referrals as needed.

Chapter 35

Family Dynamics

When a family member becomes ill or injured, there are numerous implications for the family financially, emotionally, physically, and socially. The client's family is usually his source of support, and when necessary, his caregiver. Families provide the majority of long-term care for patients. To best serve the client, CMs need to provide support and advocacy for the family, as well as the client.

To best assess the situation, understand the client's role in the family. Was he the breadwinner? Was he the caregiver to another family member? How does his illness affect his role? No matter the client's role in the family, the illness or injury will disrupt the family norms. An extended or severe illness will require modifications of family responsibilities.

It's also important to understand the family dynamics. Many families have issues that can affect their ability to adapt to a crisis such as an illness or injury. Are there family members dealing with alcoholism, mental illness, depression, abuse, or their own health issues? Is this an intact family or a divorced family with stepparents, stepchildren, and/or stepsiblings? Whatever issues were present before will only be intensified during times of stress. Continually assess the client for signs of emotional or physical abuse from stressed caregivers.

An adaptive family is able to adjust to crisis; this is important to help the client reach his goals. An adaptive family possesses the ability to:
- Be flexible
- Problem solve

- Communicate effectively
- Seek and accept help

A maladaptive family is unable to meet the changing needs of the family. Maladaptive families:

- Overindulge the client
- Foster client dependency
- Abandon other family members
- Abandon the client
- Deny the client's condition
- Rely on a single person to provide all assistance to the client
- Fail to seek assistance or ask for help

Awareness of family dynamics will assist in providing interventions and resources as needed. When necessary, make a referral to family counseling or support groups. It is also important to encourage the family to maintain as much of their normal routine as possible, to take care of themselves, and to ask for help.

Assessing caregiver support and family coping is an ongoing process. Everyone may come together initially and set aside family issues, but sooner or later the family dynamics will surface. The primary caregiver may become burned out, as initially everyone is extremely supportive, but as time goes on that support may diminish.

Chapter 36

Abuse and Neglect

There are numerous types of abuse and neglect, including physical, emotional/ psychological, sexual, financial, and medical. The elderly are at increased risk for abuse, with about 1 in 10 people ages 60 or older becoming the victim of abuse (Centers for Disease Control and Prevention, 2021). The perpetrators of abuse and neglect are most often family members, with the majority of them being adult children and spouses (Elder abuse, 2008). As CMs are often in contact with the caregivers, they should be aware of the risk factors of abusers which include:

- Mental illness
- Alcohol and drug abuse
- History of abuse
- Inability to cope with stress
- Depression
- Lack of support from other potential caregivers
- Caregiver reluctance

If the client's caregiver is identified as at an increased risk for abusing the client, some interventions may reduce the threat of abuse:

- Ensure the caregiver receives proper training and education on their responsibilities.
- Help the caregiver develop a support system, identify support groups, and locate respite care.

- Inquire about situations that frustrate or anger the caregiver and help him or her identify appropriate responses.
- If necessary, assist with the arrangement for paid caregivers or placement of the client in the appropriate long-term care setting.

Types of Abuse and Neglect

Neglect - The failure or inability to provide for basic needs. This can be intentional or unintentional.

Emotional/Psychological Abuse - The infliction of anguish, pain, or distress through verbal or nonverbal acts, such as gestures or writing, resulting in trauma. This also includes threats of harm used to intimidate a person into complying or cooperating.

Examples of emotional and psychological abuse and neglect include:
- Verbal assaults
- Insults
- Threats
- Intimidation
- Humiliation or embarrassment
- Harassment
- Disregarding needs
- Damaging or destroying property
- Isolation
- Ridicule
- Coercion
- Mental cruelty
- Inappropriate sexual comments
- Controlling behavior (prohibiting or limiting access to transportation, telephone, money, or other resources)

Physical Abuse - The use of physical force, such as hitting, beating, pushing, shaking, slapping, kicking, burning, and pinching, that results in physical pain, bodily injury, or impairment. Also included in physical abuse is force-feeding and the use of drugs and/or physical restraints.

Financial Abuse and Neglect - Failing to use the patient's income or assets for the benefit, support, and maintenance of the patient. The illegal, unauthorized, or improper use of the resources of the patient.

Examples:
- Forgery
- Theft
- Coercion
- Deception
- Fraud

Signs and Symptoms of Abuse and Neglect

General signs of abuse or neglect include:
- Changes in personality or behavior
- Sudden change in physical or financial status
- Tension or arguments between caregiver and client
- Failure to take medications (not refilling at appropriate time frame)
- Caregiver's refusal to allow the elder to be seen alone

Physical signs of abuse and neglect include:
- Dehydration
- Poor hygiene and/or grooming
- Weight loss
- Unexplained bruises, burns, scars, broken bones, sprains
- Restraint marks
- Skin breakdown
- Vaginal or rectal pain
- Abrasions, bleeding, or bruising in the genital area
- Lab results showing an overdose of medication

If there are signs of suspected abuse or neglect, ask the client if he feels safe. If not, discuss whether they need an advocate to help plan for relocation, or if urgent, ask the patient to hang up and call '911.'

Nurses are mandated reporters of abuse and neglect. If abuse or neglect is suspected or identified, they must notify Adult Protective Services. Depending on the case, the police may also be notified. Carefully document all communication and findings objectively.

Numbers for additional support

National Child Abuse Hotline at 800/4-A-CHILD.

Seniors Abuse & Information Line (SAIL) at 604-437-1940 or toll-free at 1-866-437-1940

The National Domestic Violence Hotline: 1-800-799-7233, 1-800-787-3224 (TTY)

Chapter 37

Behavioral Health Concepts

Substance Use vs. Substance Use Disorder

Substance use includes the use of alcohol, over-the-counter drugs, prescription drugs, and illegal drugs. Substance use does not equal substance abuse. The American Psychiatric Association's *Diagnostic and Statistical Manual of Mental Disorders*, 5th Edition (DSM-5) defines substance use disorder as the following:

A problematic pattern of substance use leading to clinically significant impairment or distress, as manifested by at least 2 of the following, occurring within a 12-month period:

- Substance is taken in larger amounts or over a longer period than was intended.

- Persistent desire or unsuccessful efforts to cut down or control use.

- Prolonged time is spent in activities necessary to obtain, use, or recover from the effects of the substance.

- Craving, or a strong desire or urge to use the substance.

- Recurrent substance use resulting in a failure to fulfill major role obligations at work, school, or home (e.g., repeated absences or poor work performance related to substance use; suspensions or expulsions from school; neglect of children or household).

- Continued substance use despite having persistent or recurrent social or interpersonal problems caused or exacerbated by the effects of the substance (e.g., arguments with spouse about consequences of intoxication; physical fights).

- Important social, occupational, or recreational activities are given up or reduced because of substance use.

- Recurrent substance use in situations in which it is physically hazardous (e.g., driving an automobile when impaired by substance use).

- Use is continued despite knowledge of having a persistent or recurrent physical or psychological problem that is likely to have been caused or exacerbated by the substance.

- Tolerance, as defined by either of the following:
  » A need for markedly increased amounts of alcohol to achieve intoxication or desired effect.
  » A markedly diminished effect with continued use of the same amount of substance.

- Withdrawal, as manifested by either of the following:
  » The characteristic withdrawal syndrome for alcohol.
  » Alcohol (or a closely related substance such as a benzodiazepine) is taken to relieve or avoid withdrawal symptoms (2013).

Assess for substance use disorder as it may complicate the patient's diagnosis and/or treatment of medical conditions. Most patients will not readily admit that they have an addiction problem.

As previously mentioned in Part 2 Chapter 7, The CAGE tool is available for screening substance abuse. It consists of four questions:

"Have you ever felt you should **C**ut down on drinking/drug use?"

"Have people **A**nnoyed you by criticizing your drinking/drug use?"

"Have you ever felt **G**uilty about your drinking/drug use?"

"Have you ever taken a drink/used drugs in the morning to steady your nerves or get rid of a hangover (**E**ye-opener)?"

Answering yes to two of the questions provides a strong indication of substance abuse. Answering yes to three of the questions confirms the likelihood of substance dependency.

Withdrawal from alcohol and drugs can cause anxiety, tachycardia, tremors, grand mal seizures, insomnia, nausea and/or vomiting, and hallucinations. Detoxification treats these physical effects.

The CM's role is to provide referrals to providers, support the treatment plan, provide encouragement to the patient and his family/caregivers and refer to Alcoholics Anonymous or similar community-based organizations.

Inpatient hospitalization for substance abuse is not usually the preferred method of treatment. When additional support is needed or desired, the levels of care for addiction are based on the program's structure; including the setting, intensity, and frequency of services. This was covered in Part 6: Care Delivery, Chapter 23: Levels of Care and Care Settings.

Dual Diagnoses

Dual diagnosis describes patients with coexisting mental illness and substance abuse disorders. The mental illness must meet the criteria for diagnosis by the DSM-5. Dual diagnoses are not uncommon according to The National Institute on Drug Abuse's (National Institute on Drug Abuse, 2020) review of multiple national surveys which found that about half of those who experience a mental illness during their lives will also experience a substance use disorder and vice versa. The prognosis for patients with mental illness who abuse drugs and/or alcohol is worse than for patients who do not.

Psychiatric treatment is more successful with patients who are not actively abusing substances. For this reason, the first step is often for the patient to stop using, or if the patient is addicted, to detox the patient. Additional treatment may include individual counseling, support groups, and medications to help the patient develop coping skills, build self-confidence, and manage the symptoms of mental illness.

Part 8: Psychosocial Concepts and Support Systems

Chapter 38

Crisis Intervention Strategies

A crisis can refer to any situation in which the client perceives the inability to effectively problem-solve and/or cope. A situation that may be a crisis to one individual, may not be a crisis to another. Not all crises involve danger, but if the patient is in danger, the priority is his safety. If he is admitted to an inpatient facility, he will require 1:1 observation.

If at any time the client is thought to be at risk for suicide, the CM should ask directly if he has a plan to commit suicide. If there is any doubt about the client's safety, he should be admitted. If safety is not an issue, help him develop good support systems or refer him to a support group, counselor, therapist, or psychiatrist as appropriate. Items such as weapons or large quantities of medications should be removed from the patient's access. Complete frequent follow-up assessments to evaluate the effectiveness of the interventions.

Suicide risk factors include:

- History of prior suicide attempt
- Family history of suicide
- Living alone
- Recently divorced or widowed
- History of mental illness
- Chronic illness
- History of substance abuse

- Unemployed
- Recent loss
- Hopelessness or helplessness
- Risk-taking behavior
- Giving away prized possessions
- Lack of interest in future plans

After safety is established, listen to the client to assess his state of need. Always allow him to tell his story and express his full emotions without the fear of being judged. Assist the client to assess things that have worked for him in the past and available resources. Collaborate on finding alternative coping mechanisms and setting goals, while focusing on the client's strengths.

Chapter 39

Support Programs

Depending on the specific needs of the client, support may be found in a local support group or a national disease-based program. Local support groups often meet at hospitals, community centers, and religious institutions.

Support programs are also available for caregivers. Many communities have local caregiver support groups, and national organizations, such as the Alzheimer's Foundation of America, offer support services and strategies for caregivers.

For patients with deeply held spiritual beliefs (identified during the spiritual assessment upon enrollment in case management), pastoral counseling may be an integral part of their treatment.

Bereavement counseling can aid in the loss of a loved one, as well as other losses brought on by illness or tragedy. Local hospice agencies are a good resource for bereavement counseling and will often provide this service to anyone, not just their clients.

Follow up with clients referred for support to assess the effectiveness. In addition, receiving first-hand feedback will help with the development of a list of go-to resources for future clients.

References

Chapter 31

Babey, S., Diamant, A., Hastert, T., & Harvey, S. (2008). *Designed for disease: the link between local food environments and obesity and diabetes.* UCLA Center for Health Policy Research.

Centers for Disease Control and Prevention (CDC). (2019). *Frequently asked questions.* CDC. https://www.cdc.gov/nchhstp/socialdeterminants/faq.html

Cheng, E., Chen, A., & Cunningham, W. (2007). Primary language and receipt of recommended health care among Hispanics in the United States. *Journal of Internal Medicine, 22*(2), 283–288.

Deaths attributable to the environment - data by country. (2016, March 9). WHO; World Health Organization. https://apps.who.int/gho/data/node.main.162

French, S. A. (2003). Pricing effects on food choices. *The Journal of Nutrition, 133*(3), 841S843S. https://doi.org/10.1093/jn/133.3.841s

Jacobs, E. A., Karavolos, K., Rathouz, P. J., Ferris, T. G., & Powell, L. H. (2005). Limited English Proficiency and Breast and Cervical Cancer Screening in a Multiethnic Population. *American Journal of Public Health, 95*(8), 1410–1416. https://doi.org/10.2105/ajph.2004.041418

Mentzer Morrison, R., & Mancino, L. (2015, August 3). *Most U.S. households do their main grocery shopping at supermarkets and supercenters regardless of income.* www.ers.usda.gov; U.S. DEPARTMENT OF AGRICULTURE. https://www.ers.usda.gov/amber-waves/2015/august/most-us-households-do-their-main-grocery-shopping-at-supermarkets-and-supercenters-regardless-of-income/

Office of Disease Prevention and Promotion. (n.d.-a). *Access to foods that support healthy eating patterns | Healthy People 2020.* www.healthypeople.gov; U.S. Department of Health and Human Services. Retrieved July 5, 2021, from https://www.healthypeople.gov/2020/topics-objectives/topic/social-determinants-health/interventions-resources/access-to-foods-that-support-healthy-eating-patterns

Office of Disease Prevention and Promotion. (n.d.-b). *Access to Health Services - Healthy People 2030.* Health.gov; U. S. Department of Health and Human Services. Retrieved July 3, 2021, from https://health.gov/healthypeople/objectives-and-data/social-determinants-health/literature-summaries/access-health-services

Office of Disease Prevention and Promotion. (n.d.-c). *Access to Primary Care - Healthy People 2030.* Health.gov; U.S. Department of Health and Human Services. Retrieved July 3, 2021, from https://health.gov/healthypeople/objectives-and-data/social-determinants-health/literature-summaries/access-primary-care

Office of Disease Prevention and Promotion. (n.d.-d). *Environmental conditions - Healthy People 2030.* Health.gov; U.S. Department of Health and Human Services. Retrieved July 5, 2021, from https://health.gov/healthypeople/objectives-and-data/social-determinants-health/literature-summaries/environmental-conditions#cit19

Office of Disease Prevention and Promotion. (n.d.-e). *Housing instability - Healthy People 2030.* Health.gov; U.S. Department of Health and Human Services. Retrieved July 5, 2021, from https://health.gov/healthypeople/objectives-and-data/social-determinants-health/literature-summaries/housing-instability

Picture of American Drinking Water Fact Sheet. (n.d.). CDC; Centers for Disease Control and Prevention. Retrieved June 30, 2021, from https://www.cdc.gov/pictureofamerica/pdfs/picture_of_america_drinking_water.pdf

Private wells. (2015, April 24). EPA; United States Environmental Protection Agency. https://www.epa.gov/privatewells

Research on health effects from air pollution. (2021, June 11). US EPA; Environmental Protection Agency. https://www.epa.gov/air-research/research-health-effects-air-pollution

Rose, D. (2010). Access to Healthy Food: A Key Focus for Research on Domestic Food Insecurity. *The Journal of Nutrition, 140*(6), 1167–1169. https://doi.org/10.3945/jn.109.113183

Sharkey, J. R., Johnson, C. M., & Dean, W. R. (2010). Food Access and Perceptions of the Community and Household Food Environment as Correlates of Fruit and Vegetable Intake among Rural Seniors. *BMC Geriatrics, 10*(1). https://doi.org/10.1186/1471-2318-10-32

Social determinants of health. (2020). www.who.int; World Health Organization. https://www.who.int/health-topics/social-determinants-of-health#tab=tab_1

Chapter 32

Gillingham, D. (2020). *CCM Certification Made Easy* (3rd ed., p. 169). Blue Bayou Press.

Chapter 33

Case Management Society of America. (2016). *Standards of Practice for Case Management* (p. 13). Case Management Society of America.

Chapter 36

Centers for Disease Control and Prevention. (2021, June 2). *Preventing elder abuse*. www.cdc.gov; U. S. Department of Health and Human Services. https://www.cdc.gov/violenceprevention/elderabuse/fastfact.html

Elder abuse. (2008). APA.org; American Psychological Association. https://www.apa.org/pi/prevent-violence/resources/elder-abuse

Chapter 37

American Psychiatric Association. (2013). *Diagnostic and statistical manual of mental disorders* (5th ed.). American Psychiatric Association.

National Institute on Drug Abuse. (2020, April). *Part 1: The connection between substance use disorders and mental illness*. Drugabuse.gov; U.S. Department of Health and Human Services. https://www.drugabuse.gov/publications/research-reports/common-comorbidities-substance-use-disorders/part-1-connection-between-substance-use-disorders-mental-illness

Part 8: Psychosocial Concepts and Support Systems

Part 9: Communication

Outcomes

Readers will be able to:

- Communicate effectively with clients and other stakeholders
- Identify barriers to effective communication
- Explain how group dynamics affect communication
- Utilize the appropriate type of question for the situation and the desired response
- List the various ways case managers communicate with others and best practices for each
- List the five conflict resolution strategies
- Describe the goal and steps of the negotiation process
- Apply proper documentation to case management cases

Part 9: Communication

Chapter 40

Interpersonal Communication

Interpersonal communication is the process of exchanging ideas, thoughts, and feelings between individuals. CMs must be skilled in communicating effectively with clients, family members, caregivers, providers, vendors, and team members. Interpersonal communication involves conveying information effectively, but also requires active listening.

The definition of listening is the passive act of hearing what is being said. Active listening is a dynamic process that involves hearing what is being said, as well as the processing and interpreting the words, tone, body language, and other factors to understand the complete message that is being delivered.

Active listening requires the listener to consciously choose to give the speaker his attention and concentration free of distraction, both internal and external. External distractions can include interruptions by others, telephones, background noise, or conversations among others. These can be minimized by having conversations in a distraction-free environment. This is especially important when conducting interviews with the client.

Internal distractions can include thinking about the next question you want to ask, what you want to say next, your next appointment, your to-do list, or anything else that keeps you from really listening to what is being said. It also includes any bias, judgment, or prejudice you may have about what the speaker is saying. One way to overcome internal distractions is to be present and in the moment during your conversation. When interviewing a client, address your client's current concerns, setting aside your preconceived notions, and avoid jumping to conclusions or making premature judgments.

Active listening can be demonstrated by nodding the head, making eye contact, repeating what is said, or note-taking. Note-taking should be kept to a minimum, however, so as not to spend more time looking at the computer or notepad than at the person speaking. Ask open questions whenever possible, as they provide more information, are considered less threatening, and develop trust.

Barriers to effective communication include:
- Physical interference (e.g. background noise, interruptions)
- Psychological noise (e.g. pain, hunger, anger, anxiety)
- Barriers to processing information (e.g. information overload, educational deficit, cognitive deficit)
- Perceptual barriers (e.g. prejudices of the listener formed by his or her unique experiences, cultural background, and value system)
- Structural barriers (e.g. layers of bureaucracy or other difficulties in reaching the other person)

Another important aspect of interpersonal communication is nonverbal communication, which can be more impactful than verbal communication (Bambaeeroo & Shokrpour, 2017). Body language, facial expressions, and eye contact are all forms of nonverbal communication. Be aware of the nonverbal communication that is being given to and being received by the other person. For example, a client who avoids eye contact or looks away when answering questions may not be telling the truth. Likewise, the CM not making eye contact and taking notes while the client is talking does not show true interest in the client, but rather that she is trying to get her information documented. In comparison, a CM leaning in to listen and making eye contact when speaking shows a true interest in what the client has to say.

Nonverbal communication is also important in non-face-to-face communication, such as telephonic case management. It can often be difficult for the client to develop trust with someone he has not met in person, therefore when reaching out to a client via telephone it is beneficial to use all the resources available to you.

The following are best practices for telephonic communication:
- Smile when speaking to the client as you can hear a person smiling over the phone.
- Maintain focus on the client and the task at hand. It can often be tempting to multitask since the client cannot see you, but the distraction will be evident to the client.

- Type minimally while the client is speaking. A client who hears typing constantly while he is talking will feel the same as the client who saw the CM taking notes during their conversation. Take handwritten notes or use a mouse to click as much as possible. Save the long typing for after the telephone conversation has ended.

Communication with or within a group, including a family group, is more complex than communication with an individual due to group dynamics. Group dynamics are the way members of a group relate to each other and the way the group relates to those outside the group. Group dynamics include:

Roles - The roles and identities that develop within the group, such as leader, authority, participant, follower.

Norms - The acceptable standards of behavior within the group that are shared by group members.

Conformity - Adjusting one's behavior to align with the norms of the group.

Understanding the dynamics and culture of the group you are communicating with will assist you in communicating effectively with them. For example, your client may be a 65-year-old widow with three adult children. If the group dynamics of this family state that the oldest son is the leader, the client may divert all decision-making to him. Therefore, it would be beneficial for you to include him in discussions where decisions or "buy-in" are required.

Part 9: Communication

Chapter 41

Questions

Asking questions is an important part of a CM's job. This is one of the primary ways to gather information in every phase of the case management process; from screening and selection through closure. The accuracy of the information obtained is imperative to the success of the case management plan of care and obtaining the desired outcomes in a timely manner. Without accurate information, the case management plan of care may stall or fail.

Often the same question can be asked in multiple ways, but how it is asked will influence the answer. It is important to understand the different types of questions and when to use each type. Asking the right questions, in the right way, at the right time, needs to become second nature.

Leading questions

Leading questions are those that suggest a particular answer. They lead the person answering to provide the answer that the person asking the question wants to hear. Some examples of leading questions are:

- "You haven't missed any doses of your medication, have you?"
- "You're not having any side effects, are you?"
- "You're following the treatment plan, right?"

By phrasing the questions this way the client feels obligated to give an answer the CM wants, as doing otherwise would imply that they are doing something wrong. Leading questions can generate inaccurate responses that are not reliable (Swann et al., 1982) (Loftus, 1975).

There are times when leading questions can be useful, such as when you want the client's buy-in. For example, if you need the client's permission to enroll him in the case management program at your organization, and you know it is in the best interest of the client to do so, a leading question may be appropriate. You may ask "I have your permission to enroll you in the case management program, right?" or something similar.

Open and Close-Ended Questions

Close-ended questions typically elicit one-word or short phrase responses, whereas open-ended questions deliberately seek longer answers. The same question can be asked in many ways. For example, by phrasing the question, "Are you feeling well today?" the responder is led to choose "yes" or "no". By rephrasing the question "How are you feeling today?" the responder has to describe how he is feeling, allowing for a wider choice of answers. Instead of deciding if he is feeling "well" or "unwell" he can tell you exactly how he is feeling. "I'm feeling tired, but I'm always tired after my chemo." "I'm feeling so much better. That medication has really helped my pain."

In general, open-ended questions are preferred during interviews. They allow more in-depth responses as they do not limit the client to "yes" or "no" answers, but encourage the disclosure of information. In addition, open-ended questions have been associated with developing trust as the sender appears interested in the client rather than just trying to get through a series of questions as quickly as possible.

And finally, open-ended questions can be less threatening. For example, phrasing the question as, "Have you ever missed a dose of your medication?" may make the client uncomfortable or ashamed if he has missed a dose, and therefore will be less likely to admit to this. By rephrasing the question as, "What difficulty are you having taking your medications?" you are giving the client permission to tell you about anything; including side effects, forgetting to take medications on time, missed doses, trouble refilling, and so on.

To rephrase a close-ended question into an open-ended question, begin with "what," "how," and "describe." "Why" questions should be avoided as they can be threatening, making the client feel as if they need to defend their choices or actions. Although CMs need to understand the "why," the way in which the question is worded will impact the response. Instead of asking "Why did you miss your doctor's appointment?" a better way to phrase it would be "What happened that caused you to miss your doctor's appointment?" Where the "why" question has the client defending himself, the "what happened" allows him to reflect on the cause.

Open-ended questions can be more time-consuming as control of the conversation has been given to the client. Listening closely to the response can provide valuable information to determine the client's values, motivations, barriers, challenges, and support systems. As the CM becomes more experienced, she develops strategies to redirect the conversations.

Close-ended questions do play a part in interviews and communications. They are used in obtaining demographic information such as age, marital status, and education level. They are also useful to verify or collect specific information, "I understand you were discharged from the hospital on Friday, is that correct?" "Did you report your symptoms to your doctor?" "Did you take your blood pressure medicine before you took your blood pressure?"

Closed-ended questions can be a useful tool to break a long ramble. For example, a client that is rambling and complaining about their primary physician can be asked, "It sounds like you want to find a new primary physician, is this correct?" At this point, they must answer "yes" or "no" and based on that answer you can take back control of the conversation.

Asking a closed-ended question at the close of a persuasion conversation can increase acceptance. For example, after discussing the benefits to the patient of transferring them to a rehabilitation center the CM may ask, "So can we proceed with arranging for your transfer to ABC Rehabilitation Center?"

The timing of the types of questions asked during the interview is also important. Beginning the interview with a closed-ended question may lead to a series of short quick responses as the tone of the interview has been set as rapid response, and no interest in the client has been established. On the other hand, beginning the interview with a broad question that is specific to the information you need to gather can fill in many parts of your assessment, as well as make the client feel as though the CM is interested in them as a person.

Starting the interview with "Can you tell me how you ended up in the hospital?" "Can you take two minutes to get me up to speed with what's been going on?" or "Tell me about your diabetes." allow the client to tell their story. The CM may hear information during the answer that requires more details and can ask the client to elaborate. This conversational and caring style sets the tone of the interview as the CM is interested and caring, versus strictly fact-finding.

Once rapport has been established and information obtained through the conversational style interview, there may still be additional information that is needed. Rapid, close-ended questions can be introduced at this point. Properly transitioning the interview will ensure that you do not lose the trust that has been established. Statements such as, "I have a few more questions I need to quickly ask you." or "I have a few demographic questions for you." let the client know that the interview is shifting and why.

Closing the interview is just as important, if not more important, as opening the interview. Mistakes made in the opening can be corrected during the interview, but improperly closing the interview can result in missed opportunities and/or leaving the client with negative feelings which could affect his willingness to continue working with you. Asking the proper questions at the end of the conversation can make all the difference.

Asking, "Do you have any questions?" at the end of the interview quickly shuts down the conversation. This close-ended question usually results in a "No." By rephrasing the question, "What questions can I answer for you?" you are implying questions are expected and you are interested in helping them.

A great way to close an interview where you have provided teaching or other information that you want the client to act on is to ask, "How might you use the information I have given you?" This implies you expect him to use the information or take some type of action based on the information you provided. This helps the client to make the switch from receiving information to figuring out how they will apply this information. This also gives you a lead-in to schedule your next interview where you can check in on their progress and help with any barriers they may have encountered.

Chapter 42

Communication Methods Used by Today's Case Managers

Today, there are many ways to communicate, each with its own purpose, strengths, and pitfalls. We will examine the most common ways CMs communicate with their clients and other stakeholders in this section.

Face to Face

Face-to-face or in-person communication is the ultimate way of communicating with others. It allows for the use of more of our senses, leading to more effective communication. In face-to-face communication, visual communication is just as important as oral communication. We can see the facial expressions and body language of those we are communicating with and they can see ours. The way we dress and carry ourselves plays an important part in our communication. Do we appear professional or scattered? This will influence how others perceive us and our role. During face-to-face communication, it is important to check our facial expressions, body language, and appearance at the beginning and throughout the conversation.

In-person communication allows for touch, a silent but effective form of communication. A handshake at the beginning and end of a conversation can show respect for the person you are communicating with, especially someone you have just met. During difficult conversations, placing a hand gently on the client's hand or arm can signify caring. For some clients a hug is appropriate, but should be led by the client and situation; your instinct should tell you when it is appropriate. Always ask before giving a hug. Culture also influences what forms of touch are appropriate.

Telephonic Communication

With access to a telephone at our fingertips 24/7, the ability to communicate effectively using this device is crucial. CMs communicate with clients, vendors, colleagues, and others via telephone. For a remote telephonic CM, the majority of communication will be telephonic. It's essential to be skilled and effective in communicating in this manner.

Prepare for the call

Effective telephonic communication starts before the phone call begins. Before making a call, consider its purpose. Be clear about what you want to achieve during this call. Do you want to gather information, communicate information, negotiate, obtain agreement, make arrangements, or provide education? There are times your call may have several purposes.

You will not sound natural if you prepare a script, but consider what you want to say before making the call. Know who you want to speak with and if they will want any information from you. Have that information available prior to your call. You may want to have talking points or bullet points written down to refer to, especially if there are numerous topics you need to cover.

Review any notes or information you may have access to that will assist you with the call. If this is a follow-up call, review the notes from your previous call. Also, be prepared to pick up where you left off and provide any information you promised.

Be psychologically prepared to make the call by having a positive attitude and smiling. You use more than your words to communicate. Messages are also conveyed in the way that the words are delivered, the tone and pitch of your voice, and the speed at which you speak. If you are angry, disinterested, or bored the listener will know. Make sure the message that you want to get across matches what they hear.

If you are working remotely and do not have to go into an office every day, it is tempting to not dress for the job. Studies have shown that we think and act more professionally when we dress for the part (Slepian et al., 2015). Standing or sitting up straight also helps us to sound more professional when using the phone.

During the call

The first thing you will want to do is identify yourself. The organization you work for may have a policy related to how you identify yourself. If not, state your name, title, and the place where you work, along with a brief explanation of why you are calling.

Next, ask for the person you wish to speak to or confirm you are speaking to the correct person. It is important to confirm who you are speaking with when discussing protected health information (PHI). If you are speaking with the client, you can ask for demographic information such as date of birth, account number, or zip code to confirm the client's identity. Again, the organization you work for should have a policy in place regarding confirming identity before discussing PHI. Once you confirm who you are speaking with, you can go into more detail regarding the purpose of the call if necessary.

During the call give the other person your full attention by actively listening. Avoid doing other things at the same time no matter how tempting or busy you feel. Even if the other person can't see you, they are likely to hear if you are walking around, answering emails, tidying up, or doing other activities that take your attention away from your call. In addition to you coming across as disrespectful, they will think that you are not interested in them, or you don't think the conversation is important enough to give it your full attention.

You may take notes, either written or on the computer, but be careful not to be distracted by your note-taking. Also, be aware that the sound of typing can often be heard by the other person. If you will be typing notes during the call let the other person know in advance and try to keep the typing to a minimum.

Check yourself often during the call. Keep smiling and maintain an attentive and natural tone appropriate for the circumstances of the call. Remember that the other person has no visual cues so you will need to communicate everything verbally.

Closing the conversation

End the call in a friendly tone with an understanding between both parties of the action(s) that need to be taken. Summarize the conversation and spell out clearly what was agreed upon during the call, who is responsible for what, and when you will get in touch again to check on progress. If scheduling the next call, let them know how much time it should take. In some circumstances, you will also want to send a follow-up email, so everybody is reminded in writing what's expected. Closing calls in this way reduces the risk of misunderstanding.

Email

Email is an essential communication tool for the case manager. It is important to recognize each email you send is a reflection of you and can add to or detract from your reputation. Sending an email that is disorganized and filled with mistakes will lead the recipient to think that you are scattered, careless, and disorganized as a CM.

The following are some best practices for sending emails.

Double-check the email address

It is extremely important to verify the "To" line verifying that you are sending the email to the correct person. Your email system will often fill in the email once you start typing, but double and triple check to make sure you are sending the email to the correct person. You may want to disable the autofill in the "To" line to decrease the risk of sending an email to the wrong recipient, especially if you frequently send PHI.

When replying to an email, verify who you are replying to. If you "Reply All" look at each recipient and remove anyone who does not need to receive the email. Again, this is especially important if you are including PHI. You may want to set the default setting on your email to "Reply" versus "Reply All" to make it more difficult to send an email to someone who does not need to receive it.

Specify your subject line

The subject line of your email should clearly state the topic of the email. It should be simple, short, and descriptive. If you are following up on a telephone conversation, your subject line may read, "Follow up from today's phone call". If you are sending resources you promised, it may read, "Promised Resources." If you are sending documentation on a client to another provider it may read, "Clinical on [client's initials]". It is important to note that you would never place identifying information in a subject line. Even if you are using encrypted email, the subject line may not be encrypted.

Know who you're writing to

Your salutation, writing, and closing should be consistent with the level of formality of the person you're writing to. If they tend to be very polite and formal, then you will want to write that way. If they are more informal and relaxed, your salutation, writing, and closing can be the same. If you don't know the person you are writing to you will want to be formal.

Introduce yourself

Unless this is an ongoing, established, relationship, don't assume the person receiving the email knows who you are. If you are not certain the recipient will recognize your email address or name, include a simple reminder of who you are and what company you work for. You can also use this opportunity to remind them of the benefit of working with you.

Keep it short

Your email is more likely to be read and responded to if it is short and to the point. The recipient should not have to dig through several paragraphs to figure out what you are saying. Write concisely, with lots of white space, and use bullet points where appropriate.

Explain why you are forwarding

Never forward an email without writing a short explanation as to why you are doing so. Even if the person is expecting the email, take the time to write the reason you are forwarding it. If another CM has agreed to review clinical information for you, and you are forwarding the clinical you received from the primary care provider, state it. "I am forwarding the clinical on Mr. G as per our discussion."

Proofread

Make sure the email flows and there are no spelling or grammar errors. Edit out any unnecessary content. Break long paragraphs into short ones whenever possible.

Encrypt

Any email that contains PHI should be encrypted. This includes attachments that are included with the email. Many employers will automatically encrypt all emails that go out. Others will leave it to the discretion of the sender. Be sure you know the policies and procedures at your place of employment and follow them.

Triple check the email address

When it comes to PHI and business matters, the last thing you want to do is send an email to the wrong person. Sending an email with PHI to the wrong person is a violation of HIPAA, and can result in fines and/or your dismissal. For this reason, you should check the email address one last time before hitting send.

Text Messages

Texting has become a popular way to communicate, especially with younger people. Additionally, a growing number of providers and vendors prefer to use text messaging to communicate. It is important to maintain HIPAA compliance when communicating via text messaging, as with any other form of communication. The best way to do this is to ensure you are complying with the policies and procedures of your organization. A growing number of organizations are using technology that makes texting HIPAA compliant. If this is in place in your organization, only text using this technology. Again, the best way to protect yourself and your client is to follow the policies and procedures of your organization.

Telehealth/Video Conferencing

The COVID-19 pandemic has increased the acceptance of telehealth and the use of video conferencing for appointments and communication. It is too early to tell if this will be more widely adopted in case management. As with all other forms of communication, HIPAA compliance must be maintained. Most popular forms of video communication such as Zoom, Skype, and Microsoft Teams can not be used "as is" but some do have the ability to upgrade to a HIPAA compliant version. Again, it is important to know and follow your organization's policies and procedures regarding the use of this form of communication.

Chapter 43

Conflict Resolution Strategies and Negotiation Techniques

Conflict resolution strategies and negotiation techniques are closely related. CMs may find themselves in conflict with and/or negotiations with clients, vendors, or stakeholders. When this occurs the CM's negotiation skills will play an important part in how the conflict is resolved.

There are several common causes of conflict:
- Misunderstanding
- Resistance to change
- Poor communication
- Limited resources
- Differing goals
- Unclear or unfair expectations
- Power plays and manipulations
- Personality differences

Understanding the cause of the conflict is the first step in conflict resolution. Once you understand the cause, you can determine the best approach to resolving the conflict. For example, if the conflict is caused by unclear expectations, coming together to clarify expectations must be done before further progress can be made.

When faced with a conflict, it is important for all parties to focus on the goal, rather than the person or persons they are in conflict with. It is also imperative to keep communication open and to avoid bringing emotion and/or reactivity into the process.

If the CM believes emotion or reaction is taking over, it is best to call for a "cooling-off period" where both parties can take a break, resuming when the focus can be placed back on the goal.

The following five conflict resolution strategies developed by Dr. Kenneth W. Thomas and Dr. Ralph H. Kilman (Kilmann Diagnostics, 2019) are listed from most to least desirable for most situations. Remember the situation will dictate the best conflict resolution strategy to utilize.

1. Collaboration - This strategy meets the needs of all parties involved.
2. Negotiation - Finding a solution that gives everyone a partial win, with everyone giving something up. This strategy is most useful when there is a standstill in negotiations and the parties are approaching a deadline.
3. Accommodation - This meets the needs of one party at the expense of another party's needs.
4. Competitive - This style takes a firm stand. It is useful in emergency situations when decisions need to be made fast. It can also be utilized when someone is trying to take advantage of a situation. When used inappropriately, however, this strategy can leave the other party feeling resentful, bullied, or unsatisfied.
5. Avoidance - This style avoids conflict by allowing the default action.

Collaboration is preferred, as everyone wins. Keeping the end goal in mind, thinking outside the box, and not becoming distracted by personal preferences helps to accomplish resolution. Each participant must set aside their own interest in the interest of the common goal. To do this, everyone must agree on the common goal. For the CM in most instances, this will be in the client's best interest as the client sees it.

The definition of negotiation is the reaching of an agreement through discussion and compromise. Negotiation aims to explore the situation and find a mutually acceptable solution. There are two types of negotiation: aggressive or hardball and cooperative.

Aggressive or hardball negotiation aims to result in a winner and a loser. Tactics include intimidation, manipulation, tricks, and ridicule. The aggressive negotiator makes few concessions but extreme demands. He or she may threaten to cease negotiations. This type of negotiation often fails to reach an agreement. It results in mistrust and damages future negotiations. It is not recommended for CMs, as it can result in deadlock, leaving the client without needed services.

Cooperative negotiation seeks a win-win outcome and usually results in the best outcome for everyone. The negotiator is trustworthy, objective, fair, and reasonable. This approach results in agreements faster and more often than the aggressive technique and facilitates future negotiations.

The Negotiation Process

Keys to the negotiation process are being prepared, developing a relationship with the other party, and establishing a common ground in the best interest of the client. Showing respect for the other party can be as simple as promptly returning a voicemail or email. Respect builds trust, which will enhance the negotiation process.

Communication is as important as respect in the negotiation process. It includes not only what you say, but also how you say it, how well you listen, and in face-to-face communication, it includes body language. Be clear and concise in your communication. Engage in active listening by paying attention (rather than planning how you will respond). Summarize the other person's comments and ask questions to clarify and ensure you understand his or her points.

Negotiation starts with preparation. Conduct research to understand the other person's side before meeting with them. (e.g. If negotiating the price for a product, know the competitors' pricing.) Next, establish the problems and the goals with the other party. Failure to agree upon goals can make the negotiation process difficult.

Once the goals are established, determine what areas you agree on—these can be put aside—and what areas you disagree on. In the areas where there is disagreement, begin to work toward a compromise. The negotiation is deemed successful when a mutually acceptable resolution is obtained.

Use negotiation effectively with not only clients but caregivers, physicians, payers, and vendors. Once relationships are built, subsequent negotiations will be smoother and more enjoyable.

CMs may use negotiation to:
- Develop a realistic plan of care with patients and care providers
- Obtain approval for needed services
- Control cost
- Obtain benefits outside of the benefit contract
- Determine the length of stay at an inpatient facility

Part 9: Communication

Chapter 44

Documentation and Reporting

The importance of good documentation cannot be overemphasized. A CM's documentation assists in clinical management and justifies interventions. In addition, because the RN CM's role is based on the judgment of an experienced nurse, sound documentation is required to protect CMs from legal action.

When documenting, maintain professional objectivity and document facts, recording quotations when appropriate. Opinions and biases should not be included in the medical record. The best time to document is during or right after the encounter.

We will now look at documentation throughout the case management process, as well as special circumstances and best practices. Remember documentation requirements will vary based on the practice setting and the policies and procedures of the employer.

Screening and Selection

Documentation during this phase of the case management process will include the referral source and the results of the screening. If the client is deemed a candidate for case management services, the rationale should also be documented.

Candidates appropriate for case management services may need to provide informed consent before the provision of services. Documentation should show that the following was disclosed to the client to obtain informed consent.

- Proposed case management process and services relating to the client's health conditions and needs, including the role of the CM
- Terms of the case manager-client relationship and what behaviors constitute severance by the client
- Possible benefits and costs of case management services
- Alternatives to case management services
- Potential risks and consequences of proposed services and alternatives
- Client's right to decline case management services and awareness of potential risks and consequences of such a decision
- Evidence that the information was communicated in a client-sensitive manner, which is intended to permit the client to make voluntary and informed choices

In addition to discussing the above with the client, provide employer-printed material about case management services when available, and document that the client received them.

A CM who is working for an insurance company or another payer or reimbursement source will also need to disclose she is working on behalf of the reimbursement source to provide adequate and cost-effective care. This disclosure should also be documented. Sometimes a client will fear payor involvement means medical care will be denied, or interfere with his provider's plan of care. Reinforce to the client that your role is to ensure the right care is provided in the right setting.

Client Assessment

In addition to documenting the actual assessment, document identified opportunities for intervention. Additionally, document that these opportunities for intervention were discussed with the client and/or client's family, as well as other providers and organizations, and that agreement was obtained.

Planning

The planning phase of the case management process is where the case management plan of care is created. The CM can be at risk for legal action if the plan of care is incomplete or does not meet the needs of the client. The documentation should show that the case manager identified appropriate resources to improve health care outcomes and enhance the client's access to care. When a treatment plan or particular service is presented to a client, it should be thoroughly documented in the record whether or not the client accepts it.

Proper documentation will support the CM's rationale for the plan of care developed, as well as the client and other interested parties' agreement or refusal of the plan of care.

Documentation during the planning phase should include:
- Analysis of the assessment findings supporting the individualized case management plan of care
- Client (or family) education on the treatments proposed, alternatives available, and what their benefit plans cover
- Client (or family) participation in the development of the case management plan of care
- That the case management plan of care was based on the individual client's cultural and linguistic needs and preferences
- That the client was given the information and resources necessary to make informed decisions
- Client agreement of the plan of care including goals, expected outcomes, and interventions
- Any changes or additions to the case management plan of care

Implementation

During the implementation process it is important to document:
- Services provided and/or the client's refusal of services
- Education provided by the CM
- Collaboration between the CM, client, and other stakeholders
- Resource utilization
- Cost management
- Provider options
- Available health and behavioral care benefits
- All communication between the CM, client, and other stakeholders

Again, it is important to document the client's needs and preferences were taken into consideration and honored when at all possible.

Evaluation and Monitoring

Documentation during the monitoring and evaluation phase of the case management plan of care includes:

- The client's response to the case management plan of care, interventions, and the overall treatment plan
- The ongoing collaboration with the client, family, caregiver, providers, and/or other pertinent stakeholders
- Follow-up assessment findings
- Continued review of the plan of care
- Any changes or revisions to the case management plan of care
- Progress toward achieving care goals and target outcomes
- Resource utilization
- Cost management
- Provider options
- Available health and behavioral care benefits

Closure

Discharge from case management services should be documented carefully to show that client abandonment has not taken place. "Clients who accuse a case manager of abandonment must prove that the case manager terminated the relationship unilaterally, without reasonable notice, and when further attention was required" (Owen, 2003).

Documentation related to discharge from case management services should include when appropriate:

- Reason for closure
- Client appropriateness for closure
- All goals met and closed or rationale for closing with unmet goals
- Client education received on how to follow up regarding services, resources, or funding set up by CM after the case is closed
- Copy of completed transition of care handover to providers at the next level of care (including the client's permission to disclose this information)
- Notice of the closure was communicated to the client (including the method as written/ verbal)

- Client agreement for closure
- Lack of client agreement for closure and supporting documentation to close despite this

Documentation of Refusal or Nonadherence

Refusal of services or referrals does not absolve the CM from the threat of liability. The client-case manager relationship is always a collaborative one and clients have the right to disagree with the plan or request different medical approaches to their care. As a patient advocate, it is important to consider the client's desires and advocate for a plan of care that aligns with the client's values. Properly document all communications with the client, family, physician, and other members of the healthcare team that support this, as these communications serve as additional proof that the CM has performed her duties and attempted to reach a consensus with the client.

CMs will not always be able to reach a consensus with their clients. Clients who refuse to accept accountability for their health pose the greatest legal risk for CMs. These are the clients who continuously refuse treatment options, do not keep appointments, refuse to take their medications, and do not adhere to the treatment plan despite the best-case management collaboration attempts. Without proper documentation, it could appear as though the plan of care is failing, or the CM is not doing her job. It is imperative to document all communication, and communication attempts with the client, as well as communication with the physician regarding the noncompliance. If at all possible, written communication should be used in addition to verbal as this can be easily validated.

To reduce the risk of being liable for abandonment, make it clear to the client, and if appropriate other interested parties, the terms of the client-case management relationship and what behaviors are considered severance of that relationship by the client. This should be provided in verbal and written format and documented. When at all possible acknowledgment from the client that they received and understand the information should be obtained.

References

Chapter 40

Bambaeeroo, F., & Shokrpour, N. (2017). The impact of the teachers' non-verbal communication on success in teaching. *Journal of Advances in Medical Education & Professionalism, 5*(2), 51–59. https://www.ncbi.nlm.nih.gov/pmc/articles/PMC5346168/

Chapter 41

Loftus, E. F. (1975). Leading questions and the eyewitness report. *Cognitive Psychology, 7*(4), 560–572. https://doi.org/10.1016/0010-0285(75)90023-7

Swann, W. B., Giuliano, T., & Wegner, D. M. (1982). Where leading questions can lead: The power of conjecture in social interaction. *Journal of Personality and Social Psychology, 42*(6), 1025–1035. https://doi.org/10.1037/0022-3514.42.6.1025

Chapter 42

Slepian, M. L., Ferber, S. N., Gold, J. M., & Rutchick, A. M. (2015). The Cognitive Consequences of Formal Clothing. *Social Psychological and Personality Science, 6*(6), 661–668. https://doi.org/10.1177/1948550615579462

Chapter 43

Kilmann Diagnostics. (2019, June 3). *An overview of the Thomas-Kilmann Conflict Mode Instrument (TKI) a long-term collaboration by Kenneth W. Thomas and Ralph H. Kilmann*. Kilmann Diagnostics. https://kilmanndiagnostics.com/overview-thomas-kilmann-conflict-mode-instrument-tki/

Chapter 44

Owen, M. (2003, September 1). *Termination of services: Reaching the end of your rope*. www.reliasmedia.com; Relias Media. https://www.reliasmedia.com/articles/22139-termination-of-services-reaching-the-end-of-your-rope

Part 10: Quality and Outcomes Measurements

Outcomes

Readers will be able to:

- Identify the five components of a Quality Culture
- Identify what makes a Just Culture
- Describe the role case managers play in ensuring safe quality healthcare
- Describe how case managers can positively impact Medicare's Value-Based Programs (VBP)
- List two accreditation bodies that accredit case management programs
- Identify URAC standards for case management programs
- Define quality improvement (QI)
- Describe the importance of quality improvement in case management programs
- Describe the various reports case managers may provide

Introduction

Everyone—from policymakers to payers to accrediting bodies—is requiring the healthcare industry to focus on quantifiable outcomes. With the recent trend of healthcare reimbursement being tied to quantifiable outcomes, there is a heightened focus on quality, efficiency, safety, and value in healthcare. CMs are in a position to shine in this environment by using their opportunities to directly affect outcomes from client admission through discharge and beyond. CMs in their everyday activities such as client interviews, chart reviews, and discussions with other members of the healthcare team, are able to identify potential problems in care and services. In addition to identifying the issues or potential issues, CMs are able to see the big picture and know how to create and implement solutions.

Accreditation bodies such as National Committee for Quality Assurance (NCQA), Agency for Healthcare Research and Quality (AHRQ), URAC, and CMS are focusing on care coordination, shared decision-making, and interprofessional communication. All areas where CMs are skilled and can easily take the lead in initiating organizational change to meet and exceed accreditation standards.

In this part, you will learn more about the important role CMs play in improving outcomes and ways they can demonstrate the value they bring to the clients and organizations they work for.

Chapter 45

The Case for Quality

When people enter the healthcare system, they believe they will receive safe, effective care designed to meet their needs. Unfortunately, this does not always happen. Mistakes happen. Mistakes happen because we have a healthcare system that is fragmented, complex, and difficult to navigate. CMs play an important role in leading teams and influencing others to make changes; creating a system that is safe, affordable, and meets the needs of all who enter and transition through it.

Another aspect that is becoming more understood is that to have safe, quality health care, patients need to be integral members of the process. CMs work closely with clients and their families and use their skills and influence to help clients have a voice in their care. This ensures the client's goals are understood by the healthcare team.

So do we have a safe, quality healthcare system? There are many recognized reports and studies that validate the challenges the healthcare system faces regarding safety and quality. A study from Johns Hopkins says that over 250,000 people in the United States die every year because of medical errors (2016). The study reports that medical errors are now the third leading cause of death after heart disease and cancer.

On November 29, 1999, the Institute of Medicine (IOM) released a report, To Err is Human, that opened the eyes of the public to information regarding medical errors. This was followed by a report in 2001, *Crossing the Quality Chasm*, that made an urgent call for fundamental changes in the U. S. healthcare system. It called for closing quality gaps, recommended the redesign of the American healthcare system, and provided principles and specific directions for policymakers, healthcare leaders, clinicians, regulators, payers, and others (Institute of Medicine (US) Committee on Quality of Health Care in America, 2001).

To prevent errors and mistakes from happening, the culture of healthcare has to change. This starts at the organizational level by developing a quality culture, or mindset within an organization that is integrated throughout the company.

Organizational culture is defined as the shared beliefs, values, attitudes, and behaviors that characterize the members of an organization. Keep in mind the culture drives policies, practices, and processes used to accomplish an organization's work.

Six Sigma recognizes five ingredients for a quality culture (2015):

1. A mentality that "we're all in this together"; everybody is responsible for quality
2. Open and honest communication
3. Information that is accessible and usable
4. A focus on quality processes, improving care, and reducing waste
5. There are no successes or failures, just learning experiences

Dr. Lucian Leape, a former member of the IOM's Quality of Health Care in America Committee and an adjunct professor at the Harvard School of Public Health, states the single greatest impediment to error prevention in the U.S. healthcare system is that we punish people for making mistakes (Radhakrishna, 2015). A Just Culture recognizes that individual practitioners should not immediately be held responsible for errors, but instead, each error should be investigated to find the true source of the error. It focuses on finding the system failures that led to the error, rather than blaming a person for the error.

Five Changes Leading to a Culture of Safety

1. Move from looking at errors as individual failures to realizing they are caused by system failures
2. Move from a punitive environment to a Just Culture
3. Move from secrecy to transparency
4. Move from being provider-centered (doctor-centered) to being patient-centered
5. Move models of care from reliance on independent, individual performance excellence to interdependent, collaborative, and professional teamwork.

One of the most influential frameworks for organizations to follow was put forth by the IOM, which includes the following Six Aims for healthcare systems. The framework says that any healthcare system should be safe, effective, patient-centered, timely, efficient, and equitable (Institute for Healthcare Improvement, 2019). When measures are grouped into user-friendly versions such as these, all stakeholders can see the meaning of measures more clearly and understand how they can relate these to their organizations and the care they provide.

Today there is a push for all organizations to build a culture of quality. This means quality is not a program or a project. It's not the responsibility of one individual or even those assigned to the quality department. Organizations will only make meaningful and substantial quality improvements when people at every level of the organization feel a shared desire to make processes and outcomes better every day in a bold and continuous manner.

The Role of the Case Manager in Improving Quality

CMs provide value to their organization by identifying opportunities for improvement. CMs do not promote the status quo, but rather ask questions. They inquire about the plan of care, alternatives to the plan of care, and ask is there a better way? Is this patient appropriate for a lower level of care? What is impeding the transfer? Does the plan of care align with the client's wishes? What can we as an organization do to increase adherence? The case manager asks all of these questions and more to identify areas to improve that are meaningful and impactful to the client, and therefore the organization's bottom line.

In addition to identifying opportunities for improvement, CMs are in a position to affect change. They look at the big picture and all the moving parts to see where things are working well and where the areas for improvement are. They are able to bring a team together to create and implement a plan to improve the weak areas. Finally, they are able to monitor and evaluate the results of the changes implemented.

CMs do not diagnose or treat but are viewed as influencers. By working closely with patients, families, and all members of the healthcare team, CMs can help to bring about quality, cost-effective outcomes. As a new CM, this can seem like an overwhelming responsibility. Here are some tips to help you use your influence to improve the quality and cost-effectiveness of care delivery to the clients you serve.

- **Become anticipatory and proactive.** As an experienced nurse, you understand disease processes and can anticipate problems clients will encounter. Put strategies in place to prevent these problems.

- **Use negotiation skills to effect change.** Negotiation was covered in Part 9: Communication and in Chapter 4: Conflict Resolution Strategies and Negotiation Techniques. If this is an area you are weak in you may want to obtain additional education in this area.

- **Use performance and process improvement tools and techniques to initiate change in an organization.** It may be difficult to get others on board with your ideas, but when it becomes part of the organization's process improvement, others will have to participate.

- **Develop relationships with stakeholders within and outside of your organization.** If you have ever had to discharge a patient at 4 p.m. on a Friday, you understand the importance of having relationships with providers, home care agencies, DME companies, rehab, and long-term care facilities just to name a few. By knowing who the key people are you can keep things moving, avoiding delays in transfers or discharges. This is just one example of how important relationships are to helping CMs ensure quality, cost-effective care is delivered to their clients.

Chapter 46

Reimbursement Related Outcomes

Up until recently, providers and organizations have been paid based on a fee-for-service system; meaning that they were paid for what they did. Today, reimbursement is moving towards a value-based healthcare system in which providers of healthcare, including hospitals and physicians, are paid based on patient health outcomes. Value-based care rewards providers for helping patients improve their health, reduce the effects of chronic disease, and live healthier lives.

Value-Based Programs

The Affordable Care Act established the Value-Based Program (VBP) in traditional Medicare. VBPs reward healthcare providers with incentive payments for the quality of care they give to people with Medicare. These programs are part of Medicare's larger quality strategy to reform how healthcare is delivered and paid for.

There are several VBPs. The goal of each is to link provider performance on quality measures to provider payment. Knowledge of these can be valuable for CMs when demonstrating the benefits case management brings to an organization and when developing Quality Improvement (QI) programs. We will look at a few of the programs most likely to be impacted by case management:

- Hospital Value-Based Purchasing (HVBP) Program
- Hospital Readmission Reduction (HRR) Program
- Hospital-Acquired Conditions (HAC) Program

Hospital Value-Based Purchasing (VBP) Program

Hospital VBP rewards acute care hospitals with incentive payments for the quality of care they give to people with Medicare. This program adjusts payments to hospitals under the Inpatient Prospective Payment System (IPPS) (covered in the unit on Reimbursement Methods) based on the quality of care they deliver.

Hospitals are gauged on measures of outcome such as:
- Mortality and complications
- Healthcare-associated infections
- Patient safety
- Patient experience
- Process
- Efficiency and cost reduction

Hospital Readmission Reduction (HRR) Program

The ACA authorizes Medicare to reduce all payments to acute care hospitals with excess readmissions that are paid under the CMS Inpatient Prospective Payment System (IPPS). CMS uses the Excess Readmission Ratio (ERR) to gauge hospital performance. The ERR is a measure of a hospital's relative performance and is the ratio of predicted-to-expected readmissions.

CMS calculates an ERR for each of these conditions and procedures that are included in the program:
- Acute Myocardial Infarction (AMI)
- Chronic Obstructive Pulmonary Disease (COPD)
- Heart Failure (HF)
- Pneumonia
- Coronary Artery Bypass Graft (CABG) Surgery
- Elective Primary Total Hip Arthroplasty and/or Total Knee Arthroplasty (THA/TKA) (Centers for Medicare and Medicaid Services, 2016)

Readmissions to any applicable acute care hospital in a 30-day period following discharge are counted, no matter what the principal diagnosis of this new admission is, except for some planned readmissions.

Hospital Acquired Conditions (HAC) Program

The HAC Reduction Program encourages hospitals to increase patient safety and reduce the number of hospital-acquired conditions, like pressure sores and hip fractures after surgery. This incentive comes in the form of reduced payments to hospitals that rank the worst among other hospitals for how often their patients get hospital-acquired conditions.

Impact for Case Management

The ACA's VBPs provide many incentives to improve quality, coordinate care, and decrease costs—all areas where CMs are well-positioned to take the lead. The impact CMs can have in this new value-driven care world is tremendous. Case management functions, such as assessing, planning, educating, discharge planning, care transitioning, care coordination, and monitoring, are key to meeting the quality performance standards outlined in the ACA.

Part 10: Quality and Outcomes Measurements

Chapter 47

Accreditation Bodies, Their Standards, and Requirements

Accreditation is usually a voluntary process, provided by an external organization, in which trained peer reviewers evaluate a healthcare organization's compliance with nationally accepted standards, as well as the accrediting body's pre-established performance standards. Although accreditation is technically voluntary, it is often required to be eligible to receive reimbursement from Medicare, Medicaid, and many third-party payers. Accreditation is also often required by local, state, or federal regulations.

Accreditation is regarded as one of the key benchmarks for measuring the quality of an organization. It identifies the organization as credible, reputable, and dedicated to ongoing and continuous compliance with the highest standard of quality. There is consistent evidence that accreditation significantly improves the process of care provided and improves clinical outcomes.

Preparing for accreditation provides an organization the opportunity to improve the quality of care they provide to patients by establishing, reviewing, and revisiting standards, in addition to measuring performance, and providing education. It is a chance for the organization to identify its strengths and its opportunities for improvement.

An accrediting body might review the organizational structure, policies and procedures, quality outcomes, performance improvement, client's rights, professional improvement, leadership, fiscal operations, and clinical records, as well as compliance with federal, state, and local laws.

There are numerous accrediting bodies covering case management and the organizations CMs work for, including but not limited to:

- URAC
- National Committee for Quality Assurance (NCQA)
- The Joint Commission
- Commission on Accreditation of Rehabilitation Facilities (CARF)

They have their own standards and requirements for awarding accreditation based on their corner of the healthcare industry, but the objective is always to ensure consumer protection by requiring safe, quality care. We will now take a closer look at the most common accreditation bodies for case management programs.

URAC

URAC is a non-profit organization that promotes healthcare quality through the accreditation of organizations involved in medical care services. URAC's case management standards and performance measures address the increasing demand for excellence in care coordination, transitions of care, patient engagement, and advocacy; which are all core principles of case management.

URAC accreditation standards and requirements vary based on the type of organization being accredited. For example, URAC's Case Management Standards cover both health plans and Workers' Compensation services. There are significant differences between group health case management and workers' compensation case management. For example, in group health, a patient must agree to services before a CM can initiate case management services. In worker's compensation, there is no requirement of the CM to obtain permission to initiate case management services. URAC takes this and other differences into account in its accreditation standards.

URAC's case management accreditation standards require companies to establish the policies, procedures, and structure needed for optimal case management performance. URAC does not dictate what these policies, procedures, and structure must specifically be, instead it gives the standards and allows the organization to develop a case management program that meets the needs of their clients. Metrics are designed to demonstrate the connection between case management services and positive health outcomes, which supports the growing trend towards value-based reimbursement.

URAC has education requirements as well as qualifying factors for anyone who performs case management services. Education requirements include annual professional education in current case management principles and practices including ethics, cultural/linguistic competence in the population served, as well as community service knowledge.

The standards also require a description of the types of clients served, the delivery model for case management services, and the qualifications of the case management staff.

Standards include:

- Criteria for identifying case management clients
- Disclosure to clients of the nature of the case management relationship
- Documentation of consent
- Policies to document patient assessments, including medical safety
- The development of individualized, client-centric, evidence-based goals to reach quality healthcare outcomes
- The achievement of client self-management goals and optimal levels of wellness through patient education and engagement
- Collaborative communications between all stakeholders, including clients, family/caregivers, and the healthcare team
- Guidelines for caseload
- Clearly defined roles and responsibilities for clinical and non-clinical staff
- A physician available for consultation
- Policies and procedures for patients to file a complaint
- Criteria for discharge

With these standards in place, organizations realize an increase in case management participation, better coordination, and improved quality of care, medication adherence, and self-management skills. Through case management services, organizations also realized measurable cost savings and cost-effectiveness.

When URAC conducts chart audits they are looking for several things. These include, but may not be limited to:

- Communication between all stakeholders, including clients, family, healthcare providers, etc.
- CM assessment is per organization policy and includes current health status, clinical history, treatment plan, resources required to assist the patient, care coordination/

transitions in care, safety concerns, behavioral health status, social support and needs, and input from the client.

- Evidence of client education with client involvement and shared decision-making. This could include self-management, as well as increasing the knowledge base of the client with regards to treatment and medication.

- The CM provided client motivation and encouraged engagement in care.

- Education of the client and family on our role as a CM.

- The CM plan to assure it includes measurable short and long-term goals and that these goals are always patient-oriented and revised.

URAC believes the safety of the patient is crucial and requires all accredited organizations to have at least two studies going at all times, with one being focused on the safety of the patient.

NCQA

The National Committee for Quality Assurance (NCQA) Case Management Accreditation evaluates organizations performing case management services that focus on clients who are at high risk of costly hospitalizations or poor health outcomes due to complex social, behavioral, or medical needs. The case management accreditation provided by the NCQA is based on comprehensive and evidence-based guidelines, and it is dedicated to quality improvement. The core of the accreditation program is care coordination, client-centeredness, and quality of care. It can be used for case management programs in provider, payer, or community-based organizations.

NCQA standards address how case management programs:
- Identify people in need of case management services
- Target the right services to clients and monitor their care and needs over time
- Develop personalized, patient-centered care plans
- Monitor clients to ensure care plan goals are reached and make adjustments as needed
- Manage communication among providers and share information effectively as people move between care settings, especially when they transition from inpatient settings

- Build-in consumer protections to ensure people have access to knowledgeable, well-qualified case management staff
- Keep personal health information safe and secure

NCQA accredited organizations demonstrate that they have the internal processes and service delivery structure to cost-effectively meet the needs of the complex patient and improve health or functional capability. In addition to the organization's internal processes, NCQA Case Management Accreditation also directly addresses how case management services are delivered.

TJC

The Joint Commission (TJC), previously known as the Joint Commission on Accreditation of Healthcare Organizations (JACHO), establishes quality and safety standards for hospitals and other facilities such as; ambulatory care, behavioral health, home care, and nursing care centers. Its mission is to continuously improve the safety and quality of care provided to the public.

TJC accreditation is required for hospitals and other facilities to receive reimbursement from many health plans as well as Medicare. TJC has requirements for accreditation that focus heavily on improving various aspects of quality care and safety including:

- The creation of hospital policies and procedures
- Credentialing of professional staff
- Education programs to ensure that knowledge, competencies, and clinical skills are up to date
- Continual monitoring activities
- Multidisciplinary performance improvement efforts using specific indicators and processes

At present, TJC does not accredit case management programs directly, but they do have transitions of care standards that impact acute care CMs. These are covered in Part 6: Care Delivery, Chapter 24: Transitions of Care.

Part 10: Quality and Outcomes Measurements

Chapter 48

Measuring and Reporting the Value Your Case Management Program Brings

Case management programs should maintain a quality management function to show the value case management brings to both the client and the healthcare organization. The case management program could be eliminated if it does not demonstrate the value it brings. Case management programs accomplish this by objectively monitoring and evaluating the case management services rendered. This is done through written documentation of the quality or performance improvement goals, the tracking of those goals, and steps taken to enhance areas identified as needing improvement. Quality and performance goals are often determined by the accrediting organization of the setting as discussed in Chapter 47.

Quality Improvement

Quality improvement (QI) is a systematic, data-driven effort to measure and improve client services and the quality of healthcare provided. It is accomplished by monitoring, correcting, and preventing quality deficiencies and noncompliance with the standards of care. It is not intended to attribute blame, but rather to discover where improvement is needed and to develop systems to improve.

Data is the cornerstone of QI. For this reason, the quality of the data used must be fair and accurate. Data is used to describe how well current systems are working, what happens when changes are applied, and to document successful performance.

According to the U.S. Department of Health and Human Services, Health Resource and Service Administration report on Quality Improvement using data (2011):

- Separates what is thought to be happening from what is really happening
- Establishes a baseline (starting with a low score is acceptable)
- Reduces placement of ineffective solutions
- Allows monitoring of procedural changes to ensure improvements are sustained
- Indicates whether changes lead to improvements
- Allows comparisons of performance across sites

The HRSA report goes on to state "both quantitative and qualitative methods of data collection are helpful in QI efforts. Quantitative methods involve the use of numbers and frequencies that result in measurable data. This type of information is easy to analyze statistically and is familiar to science and health care professionals" (2011).

Examples of quantitative methods in a case management setting include:

- Average length of stay (LOS) based on admission diagnosis
- Percentage of Medicare observation status patients that receive the Medicare Outpatient Observation Notice (MOON) Form according to Medicare guidelines
- Calculating the percentages of patients that have a 30-day readmission

The U.S. Department of Health and Human Services, Health Resource and Service Administration report on QI also explains that:

> qualitative methods collect data with descriptive characteristics, rather than numeric values that draw statistical inferences. Qualitative data is observable but not measurable. It provides important information about patterns, relationships between systems, and is often used to provide context for needed improvements. Common strategies for collecting qualitative data in a health care setting are patient and staff satisfaction surveys, focus group discussions, and independent observations (2011).

When looking for an area of focus for a QI project, a good place to start is with the standardized performance measures of accrediting bodies and government agencies; as these will directly impact your organization's accreditation status, reimbursement, or both. These agencies provide specific requirements that define exactly what data is needed for each measure, making it easy to know what data to focus on and how to monitor and measure that data. You can then use this information to evaluate your organization's current status, compare it to the standards, and identify opportunities for improvement.

Measuring itself does not improve the quality or outcomes. Measuring merely identifies a problem, so QI can be applied. After identifying the area of improvement, determine the desired result and the change(s) to be made to reach the result. Some of the ways to determine the change(s) to be made include:

- Research what others have done to improve.
- Set up a study to investigate the problem in your organization. Determine a potential solution. Then trial the solution.
- Study factors that contribute to the problem, then eliminate or improve them.

> The professional CM provides valuable input and insight into driving process improvement. We all know of the anecdotal "stories from the front" that identify issues and opportunities; however, without the data to support these stories, making the case for process improvement falls flat. Qualitative data, in the form of anecdotal information (or stories), helps to identify potential issues. Quantitative data, collected based on those stories, highlights the severity of the issues and provides insight into potential solutions. Leveraging data not only reinforces the process of care provision but also fosters better patient outcomes and overall improvement of health. Case management documentation is vital to achieving these goals (Gillingham, 2020).

Performance Improvement Concepts

Performance improvement focuses on the organization's functions and processes and how these affect the organization's ability to reach desired outcomes and meet the client's needs. Both quality improvement and performance improvement can be prospective or retrospective and aim to improve how things are done.

There are several measurements for performance improvement, including:

- Process
- Structure
- Outcomes

Measures of process examine what is actually done in giving and receiving care and how well clinical guidelines are followed.

For example:

- Percentage of clients screened for colon cancer
- Percentage of patients with diabetes given regular foot care
- Percentage of children who are vaccinated
- Percentage of heart patients who receive beta-blockers in the hospital

Measures of structure assess the capacity of a healthcare organization to provide services to individual patients or a community, and for managed care organizations to ensure they have network providers in place to meet members' needs.

For example:

- Accreditation Status
- Staffing ratios
- Board-certified providers
- Access to specific technologies or units (e.g., MRI, burn unit)

Measures of outcomes examine the health status of the client as a result of healthcare.

For example:

- Adherence rates
- Control of blood pressure
- Acceptable HgA1c levels
- Mortality

CM Reports

Another way CMs can demonstrate the value the case management department produces is through reports. Depending on your employer you may be required to submit reports on a routine basis or not at all. But even if this is not a requirement, documenting the value case management brings goes a long way to help others understand the impact case management has on the client, as well as the organization.

Some of the reports completed by CMs include:

- Cost Savings/Cost-Benefit Analysis
- Demonstrating a lack of results with current intervention to justify approving more costly intervention

- QI
- Outcomes measurements
- CM program evaluation
- CM success report
- Patient care/outcome reports

Cost-Benefit Analysis

Cost-benefit reports provide a summary of case management intervention and include:

- Diagnosis
- Summary of interventions
- Total time in case management
- Total cost without case management intervention
- Total cost with case management intervention
- Total cost savings

A cost-benefit report formally documents monetary savings related to case management involvement. There is a formula to calculate cost savings. First, the cost of service with case management involvement (actual cost) is added to the cost of the case management service. This number is then subtracted from the cost of intervention without case management involvement (potential cost). The difference is the cost savings associated with case management involvement.

Cost savings = Potential Costs - (Actual Cost + Cost of Case Management)

There are two types of savings: hard cost savings and soft cost savings.

Hard Cost Savings
Actual savings directly related to the CM's actions are hard savings. Examples of hard savings include:

- Transfer to a lower level of care
- A decrease in length of stay
- Negotiation to a lower rate for a service
- Change to an in-network provider

Soft Cost Savings

Soft cost savings are potential savings and are more difficult to measure than hard savings. Soft cost savings are costs avoided due to case management intervention. These may include:

- Avoided hospital readmission
- Prevention of medical complications
- Avoided ER visits

In addition to documenting the effectiveness of case management, a cost-benefit report can be used to compare costs of various treatment options or to justify coverage of benefits that are not normally allowed by the insurance contract but would provide cost savings in addition to benefiting the client.

Justify more costly intervention

When the current intervention does not produce the desired results, the CM may alert the client care team and suggest an alternative plan of care. If the cost of the proposed plan of care is more expensive than the current plan of care, document the rationale for the proposed plan. In this instance provide:

- Client's status prior to the event
- Data from current therapy demonstrating a lack of effectiveness
- Duration of current intervention
- Cost of current intervention
- Proposed intervention
- Cost of proposed intervention
- Duration of proposed intervention
- Goal of proposed intervention

Quality Improvement reports

Items included in QI reports include:

- Indicator being measured
- Case management intervention
- The measurement used to evaluate response to intervention
- Improvement in quality directly related to case management intervention

Case management outcomes

Clinical outcomes can be measured on groups of clients, such as clients with a specific disease or those requiring a particular service (e.g., hospitalization, home health), as well as individual cases. The outcomes measured depend on the setting in which case management is provided. Examples of outcomes measured include:

- Percentage of patients readmitted to the hospital within 30 days
- Percentage of patients that are adherent to the treatment plan
- Average hospital length of stay
- Percentage of clients who returned to work
- Percentage of clients who maintained hemoglobin A1C < 9
- Percentage of mothers who deliver at or after 38 weeks

Client satisfaction/Program evaluations

The client can be surveyed for satisfaction at any point in a case management program, but all clients should be surveyed when their cases are closed. The survey must be objective and evaluate the quality and effectiveness of the case management program. To receive the most honest answers to the survey, the client should be allowed to remain anonymous if desired.

The results from all surveys in a time period are evaluated to get a picture of the client and/or client's family or caregiver's experience with the case management services. Survey results have multiple purposes. They may be used for marketing purposes, or in quality assurance, showing where goals are met, and where training, process improvement, or other intervention needs to take place.

CM success report

This type of report tells the story of a client and the benefit they received from case management intervention. This is where you toot your own horn and let everyone know what a huge impact CMs have on their clients and organization.

Patient care reports

Some CMs are required to submit client reports to support the value case management brings. As care coordinators, CMs must be able to show that the interventions implemented changed the client's outcome. This information is shown in the case management report. Here CMs are able to demonstrate the value case management has had or is having on the client by recording the client's condition prior to case management, the goals of case management, the client's current condition relative to the goals, and case management interventions.

Example: At the case opening, the client was not taking his medications properly, resulting in three hospital admissions in 12 months. The CM educated the client regarding diagnosis and medication management. The client self-reports a better understanding of his diagnosis and medications and is able to verbalize correct usage of medications and signs and symptoms to report. The client has had no hospitalizations in the last three months.

Patient care reports may include:

- Justification for case management involvement, such as the diagnosis
- Desired outcomes and goals of case management
- Progress toward the outcomes
- Cost of care with case management intervention
- Cost of care without case management intervention
- Cost savings due to case management intervention

References

Chapter 45

Benchmark Six Sigma. (2015, April 2). *Five essential ingredients for a quality culture*. Benchmark Six Sigma. https://www.benchmarksixsigma.com/lean-six-sigma-case-studies/five-essential-ingredients-for-a-quality-culture/

Institute for Healthcare Improvement. (2019). *Across the chasm: Six aims for changing the health care system*. Ihi.org. http://www.ihi.org/resources/Pages/ImprovementStories/AcrosstheChasmSixAimsforChangingtheHealthCareSystem.aspx

Institute of Medicine (US) Committee on Quality of Health Care in America. (2001). *Crossing the Quality Chasm: A New Health System for the 21st Century*. National Academies Press (US).

John Hopkins Medicine. (2016, May 3). *Study suggests medical errors now third leading cause of death in the U.S.* Hopkinsmedicine.org; https://www.hopkinsmedicine.org/news/media/releases/study_suggests_medical_errors_now_third_leading_cause_of_death_in_the_us

Radhakrishna, S. (2015). Culture of blame in the National Health Service; consequences and solutions. *British Journal of Anaesthesia, 115*(5), 653–655. https://doi.org/10.1093/bja/aev152

Chapter 48

Health Resources and Services Administration (HRSA). (2011). Quality Improvement. In *Health Resources and Services Administration* (p. 6). U. S. Department of Health and Human Services. https://www.hrsa.gov/sites/default/files/quality/toolbox/508pdfs/qualityimprovement.pdf

Part 10: Quality and Outcomes Measurements

Part 11: Reimbursement Methods and Managed Care Principles

Outcomes

Readers will be able to:

- Define key insurance terms essential for all case managers to understand.
- Calculate a client's out-of-pocket costs when given the cost of service and the copayment, deductible, and coinsurance.
- Determine which insurance is primary and which is secondary when a patient has more than one health insurance policy.
- Discuss the various reimbursement and payment methodologies that are used today.
- Identify the various types of insurance clients may have and the implications for the client and case manager.
- Describe what the Consolidated Omnibus Budget Reconciliation Act (COBRA) is and who it covers.
- Identify patients that may be eligible for Medicaid and the types of eligible services.
- Identify clients that may be eligible for Medicare.
- Differentiate between Medicare Part A, B, C, and D.
- Explain reimbursement under Medicare and compare the classification systems used for different services.
- Explain Medicare's Two-Midnight Rule, The Medicare Inpatient-only List, and Medicare Outpatient Observation Notice (MOON), the implications for the patient, and the responsibilities of the case manager.
- Compare the various financial and medical benefits available to those who are sick, injured, or disabled; both on and off the job.
- Identify non-traditional resources that are available to clients.

Introduction

The bedside nurse is rarely concerned with her patient's insurance type, or lack of insurance. Her job is to care for all of her patients regardless of their payment source or ability to pay. But health insurance is a key factor in how the patient will be able to access healthcare. If he is uninsured or underinsured, his access to adequate healthcare may be limited. Even those with insurance will have guidelines to work within, limitations, and restrictions.

CMs must have a broad knowledge of the reimbursement methods available to clients to perform her job effectively. She must understand the clinical and financial resources available to her client, the eligibility criteria for receiving those resources, as well as the limitations and restrictions to the resources. When the needs of the client and the obvious financial resources available do not match, the case manager must be aware of alternate resources available to the client.

In this part, we will cover basic insurance coverage and principles. Health insurance generally falls under two categories: private, including employer-sponsored health coverage and individual policies, and public, such as Medicare and Medicaid. You will learn the basic information you need to begin working as a CM. This will help familiarize you with the terminology, principles, concepts, and alternative financial resources, creating a foundation you can build on during your case management career.

Chapter 49

Learning the Language

Before you can begin to understand the insurance and reimbursement systems available, you must first understand key terms. We will begin by defining and exploring key insurance terms essential for all CMs to understand.

Underinsured

People who are underinsured have high deductibles and high out-of-pocket expenses relative to their income. For lower-income families, this means spending 5% or more of their income on health care, while for higher-income families it means spending 10% or more (The Commonwealth Fund, n.d.).

Medical Necessity

Medical insurance will only cover healthcare services that are medically necessary. What is deemed medically necessary varies by the health plan. In general, medically necessary services are those that are reasonable, necessary, appropriate, and based on evidence-based standards of care.

Precertification

Precertification or preauthorization is the process of obtaining and documenting approval from the health plan before medical services occur.

Coinsurance, Copayments, and Deductibles

The deductible is a specific amount of money the client must pay for covered expenses before the insurance company begins paying.

Coinsurance is a percentage of the cost of a covered health care service the client pays after the deductible is met.

A copayment is a set amount the patient pays each time a specific service is rendered. For example, a plan may require a $20 copayment for each doctor's office visit, or a $15 copayment to fill a prescription. Each time a client goes to the doctor or has a prescription filled, he will be charged the copayment, regardless of whether his deductible has been met.

Most health plans have an out-of-pocket maximum/limit. This is the most the client will have to pay for covered services in a plan year. After this amount is spent on deductibles, copayments, and coinsurance, the health plan pays 100% of the costs of covered benefits.

> To illustrate: A client received a procedure costing $5,000, and his plan requires a $500 deductible and 80%/20% coinsurance (insurance company pays 80% and the insured pays 20%). The client is first responsible for the $500 deductible. After that, the insurance company pays 80% of the remaining $4,500 (equaling $3,600), and the patient pays 20% (equaling $900). The patient is responsible for $1,400 in total: the $500 deductible and the $900 coinsurance.

Appeal

An appeal is a formal process or request to reconsider a healthcare decision; such as the denial of hospital admission, an extension of the length of stay, or reimbursement for healthcare services.

Extra-contractual Benefits

Extra-contractual benefits are benefits not covered under the health insurance plan but are given to the insured due to the cost savings for the health plan. For example, a patient is receiving skilled nursing home visits for complex dressing changes and has exhausted his home health care benefit. The CM could negotiate additional visits using a Cost-Benefit

Analysis. A Cost-Benefit Analysis is a process businesses use to analyze decisions. The cost of an additional RN home visit at $100 per day is subtracted from the cost of admission to a SNF at a rate of $500 per day. These cost savings justify the advantage of continued wound care in the home.

Coordination of Benefits (COB)

To prevent double payment for services when an insured individual has coverage from two or more sources, the National Association of Insurance Commissioners created COB guidelines. Following these guidelines is not mandatory, but most states and commercial insurance companies choose to use these COB provisions to determine which insurance is primary and which is secondary.

The primary plan is initially responsible for the payment of benefits for covered services as if there were no other plans. After the primary plan has paid, the balance is passed to the secondary company, which pays according to its contract.

The following determine which plan is primary:

Employees

- The insurance plan covering the client as an employee is the primary payer over a plan covering the individual as a dependent, which pays secondary.
- The insurance plan that covers an active employee is primary over a COBRA plan or a plan that covers a retiree or laid-off employee, which are secondary.

Dependents of married parents

- If the parents are married, the Birthday Rule states that the parent whose birthday comes first in the year is primary for the children.
- If the parents are not married and both plans cover the child as a dependent, primary coverage is determined by the court.
- If no court determination has been made, the parent with custody is primary, followed by the spouse of the parent with custody, and finally the parent without custody.

Medicare

- Age 65 or older and retired, Medicare is primary.
- Age 65 or older and covered due to the patient or his spouse working for an employer with 20 or more employees, the employer plan is primary.
- Age 65 or older and covered due to a patient or spouse working for an employer with fewer than 20 employees, Medicare is primary.

If none of the above apply, the coverage that has been in force the longest is primary. If an insurance plan does not have a COB provision, it must pay primary. Medicaid always pays last.

Managed Care

Managed care is a system of healthcare delivery whose goal is to maintain quality, cost-efficient care by managing the use, access, cost, quality, and effectiveness of services. Managed care organizations link the patient to the provider and/or service and include several types, such as a preferred provider organization (PPO), exclusive provider organization (EPO), point-of-service (POS) plan, and health maintenance organization (HMO).

PPO

The PPO contains costs by negotiating discounts for services with providers as a condition for being included in the PPO. The providers with whom they contract are considered "network providers." By receiving a discount from providers, the PPO can reduce health insurance premiums and healthcare expenditures. In turn, clients' costs are covered by the insurance company at a higher percentage when they choose providers in the PPO. Clients may choose providers not included in the PPO but will pay more out-of-pocket.

EPO

An EPO is similar to a PPO in that a network of providers have agreed to provide care for the members at a discounted rate. In an EPO, however, a client is not reimbursed for services if he chooses to receive healthcare outside the network.

POS

The Point-of-Service Plan allows the client to choose to receive care in-network at little or no out-of-pocket cost or to go out of the network and incur larger out-of-pocket expenses. This decision can be made at the point of service, as opposed to when choosing a health plan.

HMO

HMOs reimburse providers by capitation, paying a fixed amount per member per month (PMPM) for contracted services. Providers are not reimbursed for the specific services provided. If the member uses the services never, once, or more often, the provider receives the same payment.

Preventive care is encouraged under this insurance structure, to avoid more costly corrective care. HMOs often use a primary care provider (PCP) to act as a gatekeeper. The gatekeeper's role is to provide medical and preventative care, and to coordinate patient care outside of his or her scope of practice. Any care (other than emergency care) not coordinated through the PCP is not covered by the HMO.

Pharmacy Benefit Management (PBM)

Pharmacy benefit management services use a number of strategies to control the cost of prescription medications. One such strategy is contracting with a network of retail pharmacies to provide discounted rates for members. They may also use mail-order pharmacies, through which medications are mailed to the client's home at a saving over retail prices.

Pharmacy benefit management services use their large purchasing power to negotiate discounts from drug manufacturers. They also develop and maintain a formulary—a list of drugs approved for reimbursement—to encourage the use of lower-cost drugs. Pharmacy benefit management services often use payment tiers, with generic drugs being the cheapest, followed by formulary medications, and then non-formulary medications.

Reimbursement and Payment Methodologies

With traditional fee-for-service reimbursement, each service rendered is priced and charged separately. A patient who undergoes a mastectomy would incur charges for the hospital room, medications, lab work, surgical supplies, the OR suite, physician charges, surgeon charges, anesthesia, anesthesiologist, post-op office visits, and so on.

It is believed by some in the medical community the fee-for-service payment system encourages the overuse of healthcare resources. The episode-of-care payment method was created in an attempt to correct this. With episode-of-care reimbursement, the episode is reimbursed in one predetermined lump sum, no matter the cost of services provided, eliminating individual fees or charges.

Two types of episode-of-care reimbursement are bundled/case rates and the prospective payment system. Prospective payment systems will be covered in greater detail in the Medicare section. The terms "bundled" and "case rate" are used interchangeably and represent a single comprehensive payment made to healthcare providers to cover all of the services the patient requires for a specific treatment or condition. Bundled or case rates are often used in orthopedic procedures such as total hip replacements, cardiac procedures such as CABG (coronary artery bypass grafting), and maternity care.

Depending on the episode of care reimbursement agreement between the provider and the reimburser, continued stay review may not be necessary for clients admitted with these procedures/diagnoses unless the client has a large variance in the amount and/or level of care they are utilizing. This is because a predetermined reimbursement rate has been negotiated for all patients receiving this procedure or admitted with this diagnosis. If the patient is discharged early and/or utilizes fewer resources, the provider makes money. If the patient has complications or discharge is delayed, the provider loses money.

Chapter 50

Private Benefit Programs

Insurance that is not funded or run by the federal or state government is private insurance. While many individuals have access to private insurance through their employer, many do not. These individuals have the option to purchase individual insurance through the healthcare marketplace.

Employer-sponsored Health Coverage

Employer-sponsored health insurance is coverage offered by an employer to its employees. The employee and employer usually each pay a portion of the monthly premium for the coverage. The employee has the option to include his or her dependents on the plan.

The employer will usually contract with an insurance company to provide medical insurance, this is known as "fully-insured." With fully insured health plans the insurance company collects premiums from the employer and pays claims based on the policy purchased.

Alternatively, some companies, with the financial means to do so, choose to self-fund their employer-sponsored health insurance. With a self-funded insurance plan, the company (employer) pays medical claims with its own money. They may contract with an insurance company to handle the processing of claims, (sometimes referred to as Administrative Services Only or ASO) and the insurance company will issue the insurance card and be the point of contact, but the claims are paid out using the employer's funds. The employer will have major input into the health insurance contract regarding what is a covered benefit, as it is their money.

Insurance companies have hundreds of policies to choose from and will even individualize a policy for an employer. It is the employer that ultimately chooses which policy they would like to offer their employees. CMs need to know and understand that all policies are different as Client A and Client Q may both have XYZ Insurance, but the coverage of Client A can be very different from Client Q.

For example, both clients may need daily infusions post-discharge. Client A's policy will cover home infusion, but Client Q's policy will not cover home infusions, only covering outpatient infusions in an outpatient clinic setting.

COBRA

With employer-sponsored health insurance, the coverage stops when the employee is no longer working for the employer. This can be for any reason including, but not limited to death, illness or injury, layoff, termination, or resignation.

In 1986, Congress passed the Consolidated Omnibus Budget Reconciliation Act (COBRA). Under this law, employees and their families (spouse, former spouse, and dependent children) who might otherwise lose their health insurance due to certain life events, can choose to keep their insurance for a limited time. The events include:

- A covered employee's death
- A covered employee's job loss or reduction in hours for any reason other than gross misconduct
- A covered employee becomes entitled to Medicare
- A covered employee's divorce or legal separation
- A child's loss of dependent status (and therefore coverage) under the plan

Employers (private sector or state/local government) with 20 or more employees offer COBRA.

If a person elects COBRA coverage, he continues to receive group health benefits from the plan for a limited time. The duration of coverage under COBRA is usually 18 months, but two circumstances can extend coverage. The first is when one of the qualified beneficiaries is disabled. The second is when a second qualifying event occurs.

Extension due to disability

If one of the qualified beneficiaries in a family becomes disabled and meets certain requirements, all of the qualified beneficiaries in that family are entitled to an 11-month extension of coverage, for a total of 29 months of continuation coverage [18 months (standard continuation coverage) + 11 months (disability extension) = 29 months]. The plan can charge qualified beneficiaries an increased premium, up to 150% of the cost of coverage, during the 11-month disability extension (Employee Benefits Security Administration; United States Department of Labor, 2018).

The requirements are:
1. The Social Security Administration (SSA) determines that the qualified beneficiary is disabled before the 60th day of continuation coverage; and
2. The disability continues for the duration of the initial 18-month period of continuation coverage.

Extension due to second qualifying event

The standard 18 months of continuation coverage may be extended up to an additional 18 months for qualified beneficiaries if the qualified beneficiary experiences a second qualifying event, for a total of 36 months of continuation coverage. Second qualifying events include the death of the covered employee, divorce or legal separation of the covered employee and spouse, Medicare entitlement (in certain circumstances), or loss of dependent child status under the plan (Employee Benefits Security Administration; United States Department of Labor, 2018).

Summary of qualifying events, qualified beneficiaries, and maximum periods of continuation coverage

The following chart shows the maximum period for which continuation coverage must be offered for the specific qualifying events and the qualified beneficiaries who are entitled to elect continuation coverage when the specific event occurs. **Note that an event is a qualifying event only if it causes the qualified beneficiary to lose coverage under the plan.**

The eligible person must elect COBRA within 60 days of the plan coverage terminating. After the initial election, the first premium payment must be made within 45 days. After this, payments are due on the first of each month, subject to a 30-day grace period. If payments are not made as stated, coverage may be terminated.

Group health plans can require qualified beneficiaries to pay for COBRA continuation coverage, although plans can choose to provide continuation coverage at reduced or no cost. In calculating premiums for continuation coverage, a plan can include the cost paid by both the employee and the employer, plus an additional 2% for administrative costs.

As stated previously, for qualified beneficiaries receiving the 11-month disability extension of continuation coverage, the premium for those additional months may be increased to 150% of the plan's total cost of coverage (Employee Benefits Security Administration; United States Department of Labor, 2018). This makes COBRA financially out of reach for many of the people who qualify for it.

QUALIFYING EVENT	QUALIFIED BENEFICIARIES	MAXIMUM PERIOD OF CONTINUATION CONVERAGE
Termination (for reasons other than gross misconduct) or reduction in hours of employment	Employee Spouse Dependent Child	18 Months*
Employee enrollment in Medicare	Spouse Dependent Child	36 months*
Divorce or legal separation	Spouse Dependent Child	36 months
Death of employee	Spouse Dependent Child	36 months
Loss of "dependent child" status under the plan	Dependent Child	36 months
Self-Efficacy	High	Provide training and guidance in acting.

*See exception on extensions previously mentioned in the text.

Note: Reprinted from, "An employer's guide to group health continuation coverage under COBRA," by Employee Benefits Security Administration, 2018, p11. Retrieved from https://www.dol.gov/sites/dolgov/files/EBSA/about-ebsa/our-activities/resource-center/publications/an-employers-guide-to-group-health-continuation-coverage-under-cobra.pdf

Impact for Case Managers

A client who suffers an illness or injury which leaves them unable to work for an extended period will often lose their health insurance when they need it the most. Clients and their families are usually unaware of the protection and resources available to them such as FMLA and COBRA. It is important for CMs to understand these options so that they can educate their clients.

Individual-purchased Insurance

Individual health insurance is purchased on an individual or family basis, as opposed to being provided through the employer. Individual health insurance policies are regulated by the state in which they are purchased. The ACA has set up the Health Insurance Marketplace (also referred to as a Health Insurance Exchange) to compare and purchase private health insurance. Although the website, Healthcare.gov, is federally run, the insurance which can be purchased there is private insurance.

The ACA has made significant changes to how individual policies are rated, and the benefits that these policies provide. All policies must cover the same set of Essential Health Benefits. The ACA also subsidizes policies purchased through the exchanges for certain qualified individuals.

Chapter 51

Public/Government Benefits Programs

Public/government benefits programs include Medicare, Medicaid, military benefit programs (Tricare and Veterans Affairs/Veteran's Administration (VA)), Federal Employee Program (FEP), and Indian Health Services. In this chapter, we review the two public benefits programs that each cover millions of Americans and therefore, are important to understand as a new CM—Medicaid and Medicare. Some individuals are entitled to both Medicare and Medicaid and are referred to as dual-eligible. In the case of dual-eligibles, Medicaid always pays last.

Medicaid

Medicaid is a health insurance program, funded jointly by the states and the federal government, for individuals with limited income and resources. Medicaid also covers services not normally covered by Medicare and traditional medical insurance, such as long-term support and services, as well as personal care services. Each state establishes and administers its Medicaid program. It also determines the type, amount, duration, and scope of services covered within the federal guidelines. The following is general information. CMs need to refer to the Medicaid program of the state in which the client resides for specific information.

Federal law requires states to cover certain groups of individuals including low-income families, qualified pregnant women and children, and individuals receiving Supplemental Security Income (SSI) in order to participate in Medicaid. States may choose to cover other groups, such as individuals receiving home and community-based services, and children in foster care who are not otherwise eligible (Eligibility, 2010).

The Affordable Care Act of 2010 created the opportunity for states to expand Medicaid to cover most individuals under the age of 65, whose incomes are at or below 133% of the federal poverty level. To be eligible for Medicaid, individuals must also meet certain non-financial eligibility criteria, including:

- Be a resident of the state in which they are receiving Medicaid.
- Be a citizen of the United States or a qualified non-citizen, such as a lawful permanent resident.

In addition, some eligibility groups are limited by age, pregnancy, or parenting status (*Eligibility*, 2010).

There are still options for those with significant health needs who have an income higher than the limit for Medicaid eligibility. According to the Centers for Medicare & Medicaid Services:

> States have the option to establish a "medically needy program" for individuals with significant health needs whose income is too high to otherwise qualify for Medicaid under other eligibility groups. Medically needy individuals can still become eligible by "spending down" the amount of income that is above a state's medically needy income standard. Individuals spend down by incurring expenses for medical and remedial care for which they do not have health insurance. Once an individual's incurred expenses exceed the difference between the individual's income and the state's medically needy income level the person can be eligible for Medicaid. The Medicaid program then pays the cost of services that exceeds the expenses the individual had to incur to become eligible (Eligibility, 2010, Medically Needy section). See Spend Down example.

Spend Down example

*Please note, amounts are for demonstration only and do not reflect actual Medicaid eligibility amounts.

A state's medically needy income max is $1200 per month. Steve's income is $2000 per month, which normally would disqualify him for Medicaid. But Steve has $1100 per month in medical expenses. $800 of this amount is applied to spend down Steve's income (Steve's income - the Medicaid income max: $2000 - $1200 = $800). Medicaid will cover the remaining $300 per month.

Once an individual is determined eligible for Medicaid, coverage is effective either on the date of application or the first day of the application month. Benefits may be retroactive, covering up to three months prior to the application month, if the individual would have been eligible during the retroactive period. This can be of significance to the CM of an uninsured client who is eligible for Medicaid. See Retroactive Medicaid Case In Point.

Retroactive Medicaid Case In Point

Amber arrives in the ED. She is a 22-year-old with a history of drug abuse who is 34 weeks pregnant and has had no prenatal care. She is also uninsured. She is complaining of severe abdominal pain and headache. Amber is admitted to the OB special care unit with the diagnosis of preterm labor and preeclampsia. She is placed on a magnesium drip.

Four days later, Amber delivers a baby girl via emergency c-section. APGAR at 1 minute is 3 and at 5 minutes is 5. The baby is admitted to the NICU where she stays for three weeks.

Amber was eligible for Medicaid due to her pregnancy. Assisting Amber to apply for Medicaid, even after delivery and recovery, will result in the entire episode being covered.

Medicaid Hospice Benefit

The Medicaid Hospice Benefit is an optional state service that includes a variety of services provided to terminally ill individuals. These services include:

- Nursing
- Medical social services
- Physician services
- Counseling services to the terminally ill individual and the family members or others caring for the individual at home
- Short-term inpatient care for pain control, symptom management, and respite care
- Medical equipment and supplies
- Home health aide and homemaker services

- Physical therapy
- Occupational therapy
- Speech-language pathology services
- Dietary counseling
- Medication for symptom control and pain relief

Individuals must elect the hospice benefit by filing an election statement with a particular hospice. They must acknowledge that they understand that other Medicaid services for the cure or treatment of the terminal condition are waived. Individuals may, however, revoke the election of hospice at any time, and resume receipt of the Medicaid-covered benefits that were waived when hospice was elected.

With the enactment of the ACA on March 23, 2010, Medicaid and Children's Health Insurance Program (CHIP) eligible individuals under the age of 21 who elect the hospice benefit no longer have to waive services for the cure or treatment of the terminal condition, and can receive both curative care and hospice care for the terminal condition (*Hospice benefits*, n.d.).

Medicare

Medicare is health insurance provided by the U.S. Government for people who are 65 or older, certain younger people with disabilities, and people with end-stage renal disease (ESRD) (What's Medicare?, 2019). It is administered by CMS. Medicare covers some, but not all medical costs and pays under the Prospective Payment System (PPS) for most care settings. Medicare eligibility is not based on income.

Eligibility for Medicare benefits requires meeting one of the following conditions:

- 65 or older
- Have a specific long-term disability (There is a waiting period, to be eligible the person has to have been receiving Social Security Disability benefits for at least 24 months)
- Have a serious medical condition such as cancer or Lou Gehrig's disease (the waiting period may be waived)
- Diagnosed with permanent kidney failure (ESRD), requiring dialysis or transplant

Medicare has four parts:

- Part A (Hospital Insurance)
- Part B (Medical Insurance)
- Part C (Medicare Advantage Plan)
- Part D (Prescription Drugs)

Medicare Part A

Medicare Part A pays for:

- Inpatient hospital stays, including acute care hospitals, critical access hospitals, inpatient rehabilitation facilities, and long-term acute care hospitals
- SNF stays
- Home health care
- Hospice care

According to CMS:

> Most people receive Medicare Part A coverage for free but some individuals must pay a premium. To be eligible for premium-free Part A, an individual must be entitled to receive Medicare based on their own earnings or those of a spouse, parent, or child. The worker must have a specified number of quarters of coverage (QCs). The exact number or QCs required depends on whether the person is filing for Part A coverage on the basis of age, disability, or ESRD. Individuals can check their status by contacting the Social Security Administration. QCs are earned through payment of payroll taxes under the Federal Insurance Contributions Act (FICA) during the person's working years (*Original Medicare (Part A and B) eligibility and enrollment*, 2020).

Inpatient Hospital Coverage Under Medicare

Medicare covers up to 90 days of medically necessary inpatient hospital care per benefit period. The beneficiary is responsible for the initial deductible and may be responsible for a copayment.

Inpatient Part A Coverage details:

- A benefit period begins when the beneficiary is first admitted to the hospital. It ends when the patient has been out of the hospital and/or SNF for at least 60 consecutive days.
- There is no limit to the number of benefit periods covered during a beneficiary's lifetime.

- Inpatient hospital care is normally limited to 90 days during a benefit period.
- A copayment is required for days 61-90.
- If the 90 days are exhausted, the beneficiary can elect to use days from a non-renewable "lifetime reserve" of up to 60 additional days of inpatient hospital care (Copayment is also required for these days).
- The patient is responsible for all costs for each day after all lifetime reserve days are used.

Skilled Nursing Facility (SNF) Coverage Under Medicare Part A

Medicare Part A covers a semi-private room, meals, skilled nursing and rehabilitative services, and other medically necessary services and supplies furnished in a SNF. To qualify for this benefit, the SNF admission must be within 30 days of an inpatient hospital stay of three days or more for a related illness or injury and be medically necessary. The client must need daily skilled care (like intravenous fluids/medications or physical therapy), which can only be provided as an inpatient of a SNF and will improve or maintain the patient's current condition. Medicare does not cover long-term care or custodial care.

There is no copayment for the first 20 days of each benefit period. Days 21-100 have a daily copayment. There is a limit of 100 days per benefit period, after which the patient is 100% responsible for payment.

Home Health Care Under Medicare Part A

Medicare Part A covers the first 100 visits following an inpatient hospitalization or SNF stay of three days or more. There is no copayment or deductible.

Medicare covers medically necessary:

- Part-time or intermittent skilled nursing care
- Physical therapy
- Speech-language pathology
- Occupational therapy
- Medical social services
- Part-time or intermittent home health aide services, if another service is provided

Full-time nursing is not covered. To qualify for home care, the patient must be "homebound" which means:

- They have trouble leaving home without help (like using a cane, wheelchair, walker, or crutches; special transportation; or help from another person) because of an illness or injury.

- Leaving home isn't recommended because of their condition.
- They are normally unable to leave home because it is a major effort.

Medicare Hospice Coverage

Medicare patients who elect the hospice benefit have minimal to no out-of-pocket expenses for most hospice services. There is no deductible for hospice care. The only cost-sharing responsibilities come from a coinsurance for inpatient respite care, if used, and a copayment per outpatient prescription drug. They are required to continue paying their monthly Medicare Part A and Part B insurance premiums.

The eligibility requirements for Medicare Hospice Benefit are:
- The client has Medicare Part A
- The hospice program is Medicare approved
- The client will no longer receive curative care for the terminal illness or related conditions
- The client's regular physician (if they have one) and hospice physician certify that the client has a life expectancy of six months or less if the illness runs its normal course

The Medicare hospice benefit covers everything related to the terminal illness, provided that it is coordinated by the hospice provider. This includes:
- Physician services
- Nursing care
- Durable medical equipment
- Medical supplies (like bandages and catheters)
- Prescription drugs related to the hospice diagnosis
- Hospice aide and homemaker services
- Physical and occupational therapy
- Speech-language pathology services
- Social work services
- Dietary counseling
- Grief and loss counseling for the patient and family
- Short-term inpatient care (for pain and symptom management)
- Short-term (up to five days) of respite care provided at a Medicare-approved facility
- Any other Medicare-covered services needed to manage the terminal illness and related conditions, as recommended by the hospice team

What Medicare Hospice Benefit does not cover:

- Treatment intended to cure the terminal illness and/or related conditions
- Prescription drugs not related to the terminal illness or related conditions
- Care from any provider that was not set up by the hospice medical team
- Room and board, other than short term inpatient or respite care services that are approved and arranged by the hospice team
- Hospital outpatient, emergency department, or inpatient care unless it is either arranged by the hospice team or is unrelated to the terminal illness
- Ambulance transportation, unless it's either arranged by the hospice team or is unrelated to the terminal illness and related conditions

Care for a Condition Other Than the Terminal Illness

After the hospice benefit starts, Original Medicare will pay for covered services for any health problems that are not related to the terminal illness and related conditions. However, the client will be responsible for the deductible and coinsurance amounts for these covered services. If the client was on a Medicare Advantage Plan before starting hospice care and decided to stay in that plan, they can get covered services for any health problems that are not part of their terminal illness and related conditions. They can choose to get these from either their Medicare Advantage Plan or Original Medicare.

Hospice Benefit Periods

Hospice care is given in benefit periods. The first and second benefit periods are 90 days each. These periods are followed by unlimited 60-day benefit periods. At the start of each benefit period, a physician must certify that the patient is terminally ill. The patient may change hospice providers once during a benefit period.

Medicare Part B

Medicare Part B is voluntary insurance and there is a monthly premium for coverage (*Original Medicare (Part A and B) eligibility and enrollment*, 2020). It pays for:

- Physician and surgeon services
- Outpatient services
- Durable medical equipment
- Mental health services

- Emergency room care
- Preventive services
- Ambulance
- Home health care*

*Both Medicare Part A and Medicare Part B cover home health care. Medicare Part B covers home health care not associated with a hospital or SNF stay. It also covers after the 100 days covered under Part A. As under Medicare Part A, Medicare Part B has no copayment or deductible for home health.

Medicare Part B has a deductible that may apply to some services. After the deductible is met, Medicare will pay 80% of the Medicare approved amount, and the patient is responsible for the remaining 20%. There is no yearly out-of-pocket limit on what the patient can pay.

Medicare Part C (Medicare Advantage Plan)

Medicare part C, also called "Medicare Advantage" or "MA Plan", is a managed care option to obtain coverage for Parts A and B, and sometimes D, through a private health plan approved by Medicare (*What is Medicare Part C?*, 2014). Managed care options may include HMO, PPO, Special Needs Plan (SNP), HMO Point of Service (HMO-POS) plan, Private Fee-for-Service (PFFS) plan, or Medicare Medical Savings Account (MSA) plan.

To be eligible for a Medicare Advantage Plan, the enrollee must have Medicare Part A and Part B and live in the plan's service area. There is a monthly premium for the Medicare Advantage Plan.

Clients who have a MA Plan still have Medicare. The plans contract with the government to administer Medicare benefits to members, and therefore must cover all Medicare services covered under Medicare Parts A and B except hospice.

Most MA plans offer coverage for things that are not covered by Original Medicare, like vision, hearing, dental, and wellness programs, transportation to doctor visits, over-the-counter drugs, adult day care services, and other health-related services that promote health and wellness (*Medicare Advantage Plans cover all Medicare services*, n.d.).

Unlike traditional Medicare, with a MA plan, there is an out-of-pocket maximum that once reached, results in no additional cost for Part A and B covered services. Each MA Plan can charge different out-of-pocket costs. They may also have different rules on how members get services, such as the need for a referral to see a specialist and/or the use of network providers.

Medicare Part D (Medicare Prescription Drug Coverage)

Medicare Part D, prescription drug coverage, is an optional benefit that participants pay a premium for. To receive Medicare drug coverage, patients must join a plan run by an insurance company approved by Medicare and pay the premium. Each plan can vary in cost and specific drugs covered.

Medigap

Private insurance companies offer supplemental policies known as Medigap to help cover Medicare's out-of-pocket expenses such as copayments, coinsurance, and deductibles. Some Medigap policies also cover services that Original Medicare doesn't cover, like medical care when you travel outside the U.S.

The person must have Original Medicare Part A and Part B to get a Medigap policy. When a claim is filed Medicare will pay the Medicare-approved amount for the covered health care costs, then the Medigap policy will pay its share. Medigap does not cover prescription drugs.

"A Medigap policy is different from a Medicare Advantage Plan. A Medicare Advantage Plan is a way to get Medicare benefits, while a Medigap policy only supplements Original Medicare benefits" (*What's Medicare Supplement Insurance (Medigap)?*, 2019). Medigap policies generally do not cover long-term care, vision or dental care, hearing aids, eyeglasses, or private-duty nursing.

Reimbursement Under Medicare

Prospective Payment System

A Prospective Payment System (PPS) is a method of reimbursement in which payment is made based on a predetermined, fixed amount (*Prospective Payment Systems - general information*, 2021). The PPS was developed to motivate providers to deliver patient care in a cost-effective, efficient manner without over-utilization of services. Providers know how much they will be reimbursed by the insurance company in advance and can either make money or lose money on the reimbursement. Where the traditional fee-for-service payment system can create an incentive to add unnecessary services, the PPS system discourages this.

The PPS also encourages efficiency. Previously a hospital may have kept a patient over the weekend to perform a test or procedure on Monday, the PPS system now incentivizes the hospital to call in staff to conduct it over the weekend. This can lead to faster diagnosis and treatment, shorter hospital stays, and ultimately lower costs.

Medicare's Prospective Payment System

Medicare's PPS determines the payment amount for a particular service based on the classification system of that service. Medicare uses separate classification systems for reimbursement to acute inpatient hospitals, home health agencies, hospice, hospital outpatient, inpatient psychiatric facilities, inpatient rehabilitation facilities, long-term care hospitals, and SNFs (Prospective Payment Systems - general information, 2021).

For acute inpatient hospitals, the inpatient prospective payment system (IPPS) is used. Under the IPPS, a case is categorized into a diagnosis-related group (DRG). Each DRG has a payment weight assigned to it, based on the average resources used to treat Medicare patients in that DRG. The DRG pays a fixed amount for a given diagnosis, rather than paying all costs related to an individual patient's treatment during his or her hospital stay. This predetermined amount is paid regardless of the actual cost of treating the patient. This approach provides a significant incentive for hospitals to decrease costs.

The Outpatient Prospective Payment System (OPPS) is the PPS used for hospital-based clinics, ED, observation, and ambulatory surgery. This classifies hospital outpatient services into Ambulatory Payment Classifications (APC). The services assigned to any APC are considered by CMS to be clinically similar and similar in terms of the resources required to provide each service.

Medicare Two-Midnight Rule

Because of the way Medicare is structured, CMS covers and pays for inpatient and outpatient hospital stays differently (*Fact sheet: Two-Midnight Rule*, 2015). Inpatient acute-care hospital stays are generally covered and paid under Medicare Part A, and outpatient hospital stays are covered and paid under Medicare Part B.

According to CMS:

> Not all care provided in a hospital setting is appropriate for inpatient, Part A payment. Therefore, when a Medicare beneficiary arrives at a hospital in need of medical or surgical care, the physician or another qualified practitioner must decide whether it is

appropriate to admit the beneficiary as an inpatient or treat him or her as an outpatient. This decision has significant implications for provider reimbursement and the out-of-pocket cost for the beneficiary (*Fact sheet: Two-Midnight Rule*, 2015, para. 5).

CMS adopted the Two-Midnight Rule for admissions beginning in October 2013. This rule established a Medicare payment policy regarding the benchmark criteria to use when determining whether inpatient admission is reasonable and necessary for purposes of payment under Medicare Part A.

In general, the Two-Midnight Rule stated that:

- Inpaient admissions are generally payable under Part A if the admitting practitioner expects the patient to require a hospital stay that crosses two midnights and the medical record supports that reasonable expectation.
    - » This includes stays in which the physician's expectation is supported, but the length of the actual stay was less than two midnights due to unforeseen circumstances such as unexpected patient death, transfer, clinical improvement, or departure against medical advice.
    - » The clock on the Two-Midnight Rule starts when hospital care begins, including care in observation, the ED, operating room, and other treatment areas. Hospital care begins after registration, and initial triaging activities such as vital signs and extensive wait times are excluded from this time.
- Medicare Part A payment is generally not appropriate for hospital stays expected to last less than two midnights. Cases involving a procedure identified on the inpatient-only list or that are identified as a "rare and unusual exception" to the Two-Midnight benchmark by CMS are exceptions to this general rule and are deemed appropriate for Medicare Part A payment (Fact sheet: Two-Midnight Rule, 2015, Two-Midnight Rule section).

The Medicare inpatient-only list includes procedures that are only paid for under the Hospital Inpatient Prospective Payment System. CMS reviews the list annually to determine if any procedures should be removed or added to the list.

The Two-Midnight Rule also specifies that all treatment decisions for beneficiaries are based on the medical judgment of physicians and other qualified practitioners. The Two-Midnight Rule does not prevent the physician from providing any service at any hospital, regardless of the expected duration of the service.

For stays expected to last less than two midnights, CMS adopted the following policies:

> For stays for which the physician expects the patient to need less than two midnights of hospital care (and the procedure is not on the inpatient-only list or otherwise listed as a national exception), an inpatient admission may be payable under Medicare Part A, on a case-by-case basis based on the judgment of the admitting physician. The documentation in the medical record must support that an inpatient admission is necessary and is subject to medical review. This requires complex medical judgment by the admitting physician, that takes into account the patient's medical history, comorbidities, the severity of signs and symptoms, medical needs, and the risk of an adverse event (*Fact sheet: Two-Midnight Rule*, 2015, Two-Midnight Rule section).

A client who does not meet the criteria for inpatient admission will be placed in observation status, which is paid under Medicare Part B. This has numerous implications including:

- A beneficiary usually pays a copayment for each outpatient hospital service he or she receives, as well as 20% of the Medicare-approved amount for most doctor services after the Part B deductible.

- Medicare Part A will only cover SNF care if the beneficiary had a 3-day minimum, medically necessary, inpatient hospital stay for a related illness or injury.

- Prescription and over-the-counter drugs a beneficiary receives in a hospital outpatient setting aren't covered by Part B. If the beneficiary has a Medicare prescription drug plan (Part D), the plan may help pay for these drugs, but the beneficiary may need to pay out-of-pocket for these drugs and submit a claim to the drug plan for a refund.

The hospital (usually the Utilization Review (UR) nurse or CM) is required to provide the patient with a Medicare Outpatient Observation Notice (MOON). The MOON is a standardized notice to inform Medicare beneficiaries that they are outpatients receiving observation services and are not inpatient. A signed copy should be kept in the patient's medical record. Along with providing the form, the information must be given to the beneficiary verbally.

More information on the MOON can be found here: https://www.cms.gov/Medicare/Medicare-General-Information/BNI/MOON.html

Chapter 52

Disability

The financial impact is often devastating when a worker becomes sick or injured and is unable to work for a while. In addition to a loss of income, they may also lose their health benefits. As a CM, it is important to understand the financial and medical resources that may be available to the patient.

Short-term disability insurance (STD), long-term disability insurance (LTD), Social Security Disability Insurance (SSDI), and Supplemental Security Income (SSI) benefits all provide financial compensation for workers who are unable to work due to illness, injury, or an accident that is not work-related. Workers' Compensation provides replacement of a portion of lost wages, as well as a medical benefit for a work-related injury. Medicare (health coverage) may be available for those receiving SSDI after a waiting period. Those eligible for SSI may be automatically eligible for Medicaid (health coverage) depending on the state that they live in.

Let's look at each of these a little closer.

Short Term Disability (STD) and Long Term Disability (LTD) Insurance

STD and LTD insurances are private insurance that covers full or partial loss of income due to an injury or illness that is not work-related and keeps a person from working. STD and LTD usually only cover a portion of the wages, typically 50-70%, and begin after a waiting period. They may be part of a workplace benefits package and paid by the employer or be offered as an option for the employee to purchase through the employer. An individual may also purchase his own individual STD and/or LTD policy outside of his employer.

The definition of short-term disability (and the period over which coverage extends) differs among insurance companies. There is a short waiting period before the insurance begins paying, usually less than 14 days after becoming sick or disabled. The coverage will then last for a predefined short period of time usually three to six months.

LTD insurance takes over where STD leaves off. The waiting period should coincide with the duration of the STD policy so that there is no lapse in coverage. LTD pays until the worker is back at work, or to the maximum amount of time stated in the policy.

Social Security Disability Insurance (SSDI)

Social Security Disability Insurance, or SSDI, is a public earned benefit, like the Social Security retirement benefit. SSDI is paid for by a tax on the employer and the employee. It is a cash benefit given to those unable to work due to disability based on physical or mental impairment. To be eligible for SSDI, an individual must be unable to perform the work they previously did and not be able to adjust to other work because of the condition. The disability must be expected to last for at least one year or to result in death. At age 65 the benefit automatically converts to the retirement benefit, but the benefit amount remains the same.

Overview of SSDI:
- Based on work record
- Funded by Social Security taxes paid by workers, employers, and the self-employed
- For those over age 18 and under 65
- Covers blind or disabled workers
- Focuses on physical and mental impairments severe enough to prevent engaging in the normal occupation or any other work
- A five-month waiting period for benefits to begin
- Approval for SSDI can come quickly if the individual has one of the serious medical conditions named on the Social Security Compassionate Allowance List. Once approved it is effective from the date of the disability.
- After receiving SSDI for 24 months, an individual is eligible for Medicare; including the five-month SSDI waiting period, which equals 29 months before Medicare eligibility

Like the Social Security retirement benefit, it can be paid to children, widows/widowers, and adults who haven't worked but have been disabled since childhood.

Supplemental Security Income (SSI)

Supplemental Security Income (SSI) is a public, need-based program that makes cash assistance payments to disabled individuals with limited income and resources. SSI is financed by general revenues collected by the Treasury Department. The disability criteria are the same as for SSDI. Individuals eligible for SSI are also usually eligible for Medicaid.

Benefit types:
- Age (65 and older) and meet financial criteria (No disability required)
- Disability (any age, includes children)
- Blindness (any age, includes children)

The chart below is an easy reference of the most common public benefits programs.

	Medicare	Medicaid	SSDI	SSI
Benefit type	Medical	Medical	Cash benefit	Cash benefit
Benefits based on	Earnings	Need	Earnings	Need
Financed by	Employer and wage contributions	General revenues	Employer and wage contributions	General revenues
Income/resource limit for eligibility	No limit	Income and resource limits	No limit	Income and resource limits
Work credits required	Yes	No	Yes	No
Basis for benefit amount	N/A	N/A	Average lifetime earnings	Federal and state laws

Table 52-1. Common benefit programs.

Comparison of Public Benefit Programs

Workers' Compensation

Workers' Compensation laws protect employees who are injured or disabled on the job. They are designed to provide fixed monetary awards, eliminating the need for litigation. Benefits include both medical costs and lost wages, and are awarded to the worker regardless of who was at fault for the accident.

The employer is 100% responsible for paying for Workers' Compensation insurance. The employer is also responsible for filing the First Report of Injury with the insurance carrier, and the state workers' compensation agency if required. In addition to covering injured and disabled workers, workers' compensation also provides benefits for the dependents of workers killed by work-related accidents or illnesses.

Workers' Compensation regulations vary from state to state, and state mandates take precedence over the financial status or will of the employer. Federal statutes are limited to federal employees or those workers who are employed in some significant aspect of interstate commerce.

Workers' Compensation pays for:

- Medical care that is considered "reasonable and customary" for work-related injuries, beginning immediately after the injury occurs
- Temporary disability benefits
- Permanent partial and permanent total disability benefits to workers who have lasting consequences of disabilities caused on the job
- Rehabilitation and training benefits for those unable to return to pre-injury careers
- Benefits to survivors of workers who die of work-related causes

Workers' Compensation always pays primary to short-term disability (STD), long-term disability (LTD), and Social Security Disability Insurance (SSDI).

The Disability Comparison chart provides a quick overview of the differences between the types of disability coverage we discussed.

	WC	STD	LTD	SSDI	SSI
Wage replacement	Yes, a portion	Yes, a portion	Yes, a portion	Yes, amount depends on work record	Yes, a portion
Medical benefit	Yes, for a work-related injury	No	No	Medicare is available after 24 months of receiving SSDI	Medicaid may be immediately available, depending on state
Work-related	Yes	Covers non-work-related injury, accident, or illness	Covers non-work-related injury, accident, or illness	Covers non-work-related injury, accident, or illness	Covers non-work-related injury, accident, or illness
Paid by	Employer	Employer, employee, or both	Employer, employee, or both	Funded by Social Security taxes paid by workers, employers, and the self-employed	Government
Waiting period	No (depends on state – there can be 7-day waiting period)	Yes, usually 7-30 days (and ends 90-180 days after day of disability)	Yes, LTD usually begins after STD ends	5-month waiting period	5-month waiting period

Table 52-2. Disability Comparison Chart

Part 11: Reimbursement Methods and Managed Care Principles

Chapter 53

Additional Financial Resources

A significant injury or the diagnosis of a serious or terminal illness can be financially devastating for an individual and his or her family. Health insurance, if available, will only cover a portion of the expenses. There are co-pays, deductibles, and coinsurances that must be paid. In addition, traditional health insurance only covers medical expenses. Home modifications, caregivers, healthy meals, and transportation to doctor appointments and treatments are not covered by insurance.

Mounting medical bills can quickly deplete a person's entire life savings. Sometimes the patient will not be able to work due to his condition. This can lead to loss of health insurance just when he needs it the most. Loss of wages and insurance is not an issue for those who are retired, but living on a fixed income can make unexpected expenses related to a serious illness or injury a hardship.

There will be times when CMs will need to refer clients to resources beyond their health benefits. Therefore, it is important to be aware of the additional resources available to assist clients. We will look at some of the most widely available resources, but it is important to note additional resources will be available depending on the location of the patient and their individual circumstances.

Family

Families often supply a portion of the resources for the client. The culture of the family may influence how receptive they are to assist a family member, both financially and in a caregiver role. Some cultures have a strong belief it is the family's responsibility to care for their family members. This not only includes the nuclear family, but also extended family members. Other cultures believe it is society, the government, or paid caregivers' role to care for people, including members of their family.

Family support may include meals, transportation, caregiving, housekeeping as well as financial support. CMs can facilitate a family meeting where the needs of the client are discussed. Encourage each family member to participate on some level and not let one family member take on the majority of the responsibility. Each family member's abilities and resources should be taken into consideration.

Long-Term Care Insurance

Long-term care (LTC) services assist people with ADLs and can be provided at home, in the community, or a facility. Facilities that provide LTC include nursing homes and assisted living facilities. Traditional insurance and Medicare do not pay for LTC. An LTC policy may offset some or all of the cost of LTC. These policies vary widely, but usually have a limit on the dollar amount or number of years one can receive the benefit.

Some policies cover care in the client's home, while others only cover care in a facility. Depending on the LTC insurance policy, the patient may be able to hire independent providers or family members to care for him. Other companies require the client to use a certified agency or licensed providers. Some of the services that may be covered include adult daycare, home care, home modifications, assisted living, and nursing home.

Medicaid Waiver Programs

Medicaid covers LTC for people who have exhausted their resources. Nearly two-thirds of nursing home residents in the United States have Medicaid coverage (Hamilton, 2012).

Medicaid Waiver programs provide LTC services at home and in the community to people who would otherwise be in an institution, nursing home, or hospital. Prior to the waivers, the federal Medicaid program only paid for LTC services provided in an institution.

Waiver programs can provide a combination of standard medical services and non-medical services. Standard services include, but are not limited to case management, homemaker, home health aide, personal care, adult day health services, habilitation (both day and residential), and respite care. States can also propose other services that may assist in diverting and/or transitioning individuals from institutional settings into their homes and communities.

The Katie Beckett Waiver enables severely disabled children and adults to be cared for at home, and to be eligible for Medicaid based on the affected individual's income and assets alone. Before the Katie Beckett Waiver, the income of legally liable relatives was counted when the individual was cared for at home.

Disease Based Programs

Numerous disease-based organizations provide a variety of types of support to patients with specific diseases. For a breast cancer diagnosis alone, there are resources for free wigs, scarves, and house cleaning. The American Cancer Society offers clients assistance with lodging when traveling for care away from home, local transportation to and from treatments and appointments, and online support groups, along with many other resources.

The American Kidney Fund provides assistance with health insurance premiums, transportation costs, prescription medication, and other expenses related to care. The Alzheimer's Foundation of America offers support services and strategies for caregivers. The ALS Association has online resources and local chapters for support and resources.

The HealthWell Foundation assists patients in covering copayments, health care premiums, and some deductibles for a variety of diseases. Their list of disease funds available is constantly changing so it is best to check their website frequently. https://www.healthwellfoundation.org/disease-funds/?fund_status%5b%5d=open&fund_status%5b%5d=re-enrollment

The Leukemia & Lymphoma Society has a co-pay assistance program, a financial assistance program for CML patients, a patient travel assistance program, as well as other financial assistance.

The CancerCare Copay Assistance Foundation assists cancer patients with co-payments for chemotherapy and targeted treatment drugs. They help 180,000 people each year afford insurance copayments. The diagnoses and products covered are open and close based on funding.

The Patient Access Network (PAN) helps patients cover the out-of-pocket costs for the treatment of dozens of rare and life-threatening diseases. The Foundation updates its website daily with the funding status and availability of financial help within each of its many programs.

CMs can do a search on the internet for national and local programs available to their specific patients. It is also good to network with other case managers to share resources found. Many programs are reliant on funding and may open and close as funding is available

Community and National Resources

Community resources, fraternal organizations, and religious organizations frequently offer a variety of resources ranging from food pantries to building wheelchair ramps.

The Area Agency on Aging assists clients 60 and older and those with disabilities to live in their homes and communities for as long as possible. They do this by providing services such as transportation, caregiver support, adult daycare, meals on wheels, homemakers, home health, personal care, and respite care among other services.

People with limited income may have to choose between food and their medications. Nearly all communities have local food banks to provide nutritious food for needy members of the community. In addition, many drugstores and grocery stores chains have programs allowing patients to refill their generic medications for free or a nominal fee. Some pharmaceutical companies offer pharmacy assistance programs, through which some of their medications can be obtained by uninsured or low-income individuals at a discount or no cost. Many states also have pharmacy assistance programs for seniors and other qualifying individuals.

Other community resources include:
- Charity organizations (United Way)
- Service organizations (Rotary, Elks, Lions Club)
- Make-A-Wish
- American Association of Retired Persons (AARP)
- Public Health Departments

Special Needs Trusts

A trust is a relationship between three parties: a donor who contributes the funds for the trust, a trustee who manages and administers the funds according to the donor's wishes, and a beneficiary who receives the funds. A special needs trust (SNT) is designed for beneficiaries who are disabled, either physically or mentally. SNTs can be tailored to meet the unique circumstances of each family.

Types of SNTs include General Support and Supplemental Care. The General Support SNT is designed to be the primary or sole source of benefits for the beneficiary. This type of trust is considered an available resource of the beneficiary and can make him or her ineligible for needs-based benefits. The Supplemental Care SNT is designed as a secondary source of benefits for the beneficiary after governmental benefits have been exhausted. A properly prepared Supplemental Care SNT will allow the beneficiary to be eligible for need-based government benefits, such as Medicaid and Supplemental Security Income, while still receiving funds from the trust.

Accelerated Death Benefit

Some life insurance policies have an accelerated death benefit (ADB) rider, allowing an insured person with a terminal illness to use some of the policy's benefits before dying. The ADB is deducted from the amount the beneficiaries receive at death. There are restrictions on how the money can be used; generally, it can be used for long-term care and medical expenses.

Viatical Settlements

A life insurance policy is personal property, meaning it can be sold. A viatical settlement sells the life insurance policy of a person with a terminal or life-threatening illness and a life expectancy of fewer than five years to a third party for cash. There are no restrictions on how this money can be used. The purchasing party then becomes the beneficiary and takes responsibility for paying the premium.

The insured is normally paid between 50-80% of the face value of the policy. This amount is dependent on several factors, such as life expectancy, current interest rates, and the cost of paying the premium.

Due to HIPAA protections, the money received from a viatical settlement is usually free from federal income tax. On the other hand, earnings may impact eligibility for some means-based programs such as Medicaid.

Reverse Mortgages

A reverse mortgage may be an option for a patient who is a homeowner and age 62 or older. Under a reverse mortgage, the patient borrows against his or her home's value without having to leave the home or make payments.

The funds can be distributed by:
- Lump-sum
- Fixed monthly installments
- Line of credit

The payment structure of the proceeds may impact Medicaid eligibility. The line of credit is the most popular choice and often is not considered an asset when determining Medicaid eligibility.

The amount of money received through a reverse mortgage is determined by the home's value, the age of the borrower, and current interest rates. There are no restrictions on how the money can be used. The loan does not have to be repaid until the last borrower dies, sells the house, or moves out.

A reverse mortgage is not for everyone. Both spouses must be 62 or older to be listed on the reverse mortgage deed. If only one spouse is listed, and he or she dies first, the surviving spouse must repay the loan in full or be evicted.

Aunt Bertha

Finding resources for patients can be one of the most time-consuming parts of being a CM. If you are lucky, your place of employment will have a database you can use. But what if you work as a telephonic CM and your clients are in another state? How do you find out about resources available in their local area? What about the inpatient CM working in Florida, whose patients are often snowbirds returning north after discharge? There is now an online resource to help called Aunt Bertha.

Aunt Bertha helps you find information on federal, state, county, city, and charitable programs available to your patients by zip code. You can find this information at findhelp.org.

Take the Foundations of Case Management Course and Get Nursing CE Credit!

Did you know that there is a course you can take that follows along with this book? After completing the course you will receive a certificate of completion from the Case Management Institute that you can proudly add to your resume and LinkedIn profile.

In addition, the course provides you with:

- Nursing CE
- Assignments to solidify your learning
- Individualized instructor support and feedback on your assignments to ensure you "get it"
- Access to the best case management instructors in the industry!

For more information go to:

CaseManagementInstitute.com

References

Chapter 49

The Commonwealth Fund. (n.d.). *61 million are either uninsured or underinsured.* Commonwealthfund.org. Retrieved July 8, 2021, from https://www.commonwealthfund.org/publications/newsletter-article/61-million-are-either-uninsured-or-underinsured

Chapter 50

Employee Benefits Security Administration; United States Department of Labor. (2018). An Employer's Guide to Group Health Continuation Coverage Under COBRA. In *U.S. Department of Labor* (p. 9). https://www.dol.gov/sites/dolgov/files/ebsa/about-ebsa/our-activities/resource-center/publications/an-employers-guide-to-group-health-continuation-coverage-under-cobra.pdf

Chapter 51

Eligibility. (2010). Medicaid.gov; Centers for Medicare & Medicaid Services. https://www.medicaid.gov/medicaid/eligibility/index.html

Fact sheet: Two-Midnight Rule. (2015, October 30). CMS.gov; U.S. Centers for Medicare & Medicaid Services. https://www.cms.gov/newsroom/fact-sheets/fact-sheet-two-midnight-rule-0

Hospice benefits. (n.d.). Medicaid.gov; Centers for Medicare & Medicaid Services. Retrieved July 8, 2021, from https://www.medicaid.gov/medicaid/benefits/hospice-benefits/index.html

Medicare Advantage Plans cover all Medicare services. (n.d.). Medicare.gov; U.S. Centers for Medicare & Medicaid Services. Retrieved July 8, 2021, from https://www.medicare.gov/what-medicare-covers/what-medicare-health-plans-cover/medicare-advantage-plans-cover-all-medicare-services

Original Medicare (Part A and B) eligibility and enrollment. (2020, July 8). www.cms.gov; U.S. Centers for Medicare & Medicaid Services. https://www.cms.gov/Medicare/Eligibility-and-Enrollment/OrigMedicarePartABEligEnrol

Prospective Payment Systems - general information. (2021, February 24). CMS.gov; U.S. Centers for Medicare & Medicaid Services. https://www.cms.gov/Medicare/Medicare-Fee-for-Service-Payment/ProspMedicareFeeSvcPmtGen

What is Medicare Part C? (2014, August 11). HHS.gov; U.S. Department of Health & Human Services. https://www.hhs.gov/answers/medicare-and-medicaid/what-is-medicare-part-c/index.html

What's Medicare Supplement Insurance (Medigap)? (2019). Medicare.gov; U.S. Centers for Medicare & Medicaid Services. https://www.medicare.gov/supplements-other-insurance/whats-medicare-supplement-insurance-medigap

What's Medicare? (2019). Medicare.gov; U.S. Centers for Medicare & Medicaid Services. https://www.medicare.gov/what-medicare-covers/your-medicare-coverage-choices/whats-medicare

Chapter 53

Hamilton, T. E. (2012). Reducing avoidable hospitalizations among Nursing Facility residents. In *CMS.gov* (p. 2). Centers for Medicare & Medicaid Services. https://www.cms.gov/Medicare/Provider-Enrollment-and-Certification/SurveyCertificationGenInfo/Downloads/SC12-23-Opportunity-to-Reduce-Need-for-Hospitalizations.pdf

Appendix

Abbreviations

ACA	Affordable Care Act
APC	Ambulatory Payment Classification
CM	Case Manager
CMG	Case Mix Group
CMS	Centers for Medicare and Medicaid Services
COB	Coordination of Benefits
COBRA	Consolidated Omnibus Budget Reconciliation Act
DRG	Diagnosis Related Group
ERR	Excess Readmission Ratio
EPO	Exclusive Provider Organization
FMLA	Family and Medical Leave Act
HAC	Hospital Acquired Conditions
HRR	Hospital Readmission Reduction
HHRG	Home Health Resource Group
IHS	Indian Health Service
IPPS	Inpatient Prospective Payment System
LTC	Long-term Care
LTD	Long-Term Disability
MDS	Minimum Data Set
MOON	Medicare Outpatient Observation Notice
OASIS	Outcome and Assessment Information Set - used by Home Health
OPPS	Outpatient Prospective Payment System
POS	Point-Of-Service
PPS	Prospective Payment System
PPO	Preferred Provider Organization
RUG	Resource Utilization Group
SDH	Social Determinants of Health
STD	Short-Term Disability
SSI	Supplemental Security Income
SSDI	Social Security Disability Insurance
SNF	Skilled Nursing Facility
VA	Veterans Administration
VBP	Value-Based Program

Index

Made in the USA
Coppell, TX
03 April 2022

75934713R00181